PREVENTION OF DEMENTIA

Prevent Cognitive Decline And Restore Your Brain Health

By

Selva Sugunendran

CEng, MIEE, MCMI, CHt, MIMDHA,MBBNLP, MABNLP

#1 Best Selling Author, Speaker & Coach

Medical Disclaimer: The author of this book is a competent, experienced writer. He has taken every opportunity to ensure all information presented here is correct and up to date at the time of writing. No documentation within this book has been evaluated by the Food and Drug Administration, and no documentation should be used to diagnose, treat, cure, or prevent any disease.

Any information is to be used for educational and information purposes only. It should never be substituted for the medical advice from your own doctor or other health care professionals.

We do not dispense medical advice, prescribe drugs or diagnose any illnesses with our literature.

The author and publisher are not responsible or liable for any self or third-party diagnosis made by visitors based upon the content in this book. The author or publisher does not in any way endorse any commercial products or services linked from other websites to this book.

Please, always consult your doctor or health care specialist if you are in any way concerned about your physical wellbeing.

FOREWORD

"My dementia hasn't just affected me - it's affected my friends and family, too"- **Gerry Anderson**

"The goal of my diet-style is eating for optimal health and longevity. What greater benefit could there be than living healthfully and actively into old age with no dependence on medications and almost no risk of heart disease, diabetes or dementia?" - **Joel Fuhrman**

"My grandmother has dementia, and my mother is looking after her as her primary caregiver. Seeing their relationship has had a profound impact, seeing how tough it is for both of them and seeing how the roles change and how my mother has gone from being a daughter to being the mother"- **Felicity Jones**

I can relate with Felicity Jones' experience. Allow me to introduce you to Mary, a 73 years old neighbour of mine. Mary used to have her families around every weekend. She would play with her grandchildren. She had a very beautiful smile that it is always a scene to behold when she teases her beautiful grandchildren while they all have fun. Mary is a devoted Christian and would go to church with all her children on Sundays. Mary isn't just the pride of her family, but also that of the neighbourhood. Years after, things began to change gradually. Mary began to suffer from memory loss, she would forget the names of her grandchildren at times. It was just a subtle decline in her cognitive capabilities. Her children ignorantly related it to old age. And then, suddenly, it worsensed. Mary needed help with every aspect of normal living. Her vision, memory, reasoning declined to an extent that she kept asking the same question over and over again. One had to be very observant to know when she wanted to poo. Mary couldn't play with her granddaughter anymore. Sometimes she would send them away taking them for total strangers. She couldn't keep track of the date, and going to church was out of the question. Her family no longer visited regularly. She was no longer the pride that she used to be.

What happened with Mary is a condition called Dementia. Dementia is the progressive decline in the cognitive function, including all aspects of perception, thinking, remembering and reasoning. This condition is termed progressive as it leads to the deterioration of the mind, affecting an individual's ability to concentrate on daily tasks. The memory is often affected which results in the patient to forget people, dates and events that are recent to them. In addition their behaviour becomes erratic and the irability to control feelings is also affected. All in all their personality sems noticeably different than is usual for them.

According to the World Health Organization (WHO), around 50 million people suffer from dementia around the World. 60% out of these individuals are from low-to-middle income countries. The estimated general population aged 60 and over with dementia at a given time is between 5 to 8 per every 100 people. Therefore, an increasingly ageing population further increases the risk of dementia in future years.

Every year WHO records more than 10 million new cases of dementia from around the world. This means one new person develops dementia every 3 seconds. In 2030, the number of people who suffer from dementia is estimated to rise up to 82 million and in 2050 up to 152 million. Majority of these individuals are expected to be from the developing countries of the World.

Dementia costs a lot for the world economy. In 2015 it cost the world around $818 billion and it is estimated to rise up to 2 trillion by 2030.

As of today, Dementia doesn't have a cure, but it can be prevented. Dementia isn't a normal part of ageing as believed by some people. However, statistics show that "The older you are, the more likely you are to be affected by dementia. Approximately 1 in 10 people aged 65-69 have dementia. Nearly 1 in 2 people aged 85-89 have dementia." Preventing dementia is suggested to be possible to a certain extent if interventions are created to build up resilience and healthier lifestyles. Adopting a healthy lifestyle may help to ward off dementia as it does for other diseases.

Most people suffer a great deal from the lack of information and at the right time. The urgent need to educate and inform people on how to prevent dementia resulted in the book titled "Prevention of Dementia - Prevent Cognitive Decline and Restore your Brian Health" According to many studies carried out, there are certainly several ways to prevent or at least delay the onset of dementia. As explained by Selva Sugunendran in his fact- filled and based on the latest research, recognizing the risk factors and working on the modifiable factors can reduce the prevalence. This book is written just for that. In my opinion, this book is a must have for every family. If Mary's family had been informed and educated with the contents of this book, maybe, they would still be living with pride and happiness which charecterised them previously.

Prevention is said to be better than cure. Get a copy of this book and be certain to not let lack of knowledge of the latest reseach depreciate the effectiveness of a prominent member in your family.

Joseph Manning

DEDICATION

This book is dedicated to those who wish to learn what they could do to prevent the onset of Dementia as well as for those who have just been diagnosed with or have symptoms of Dementia and to their families, to show that there is hope.

ABOUT THE AUTHOR

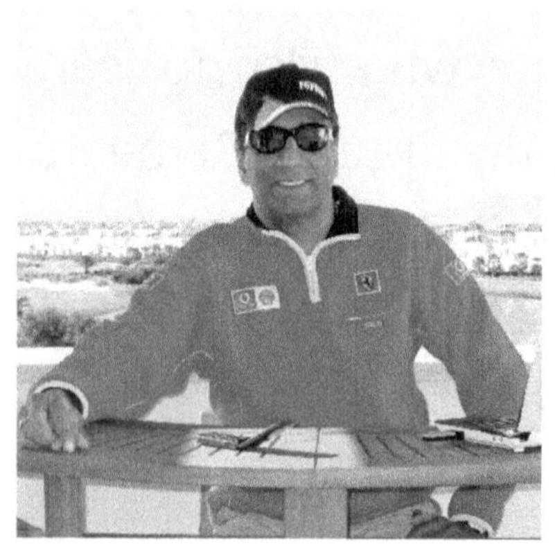 **S**elva Sugunendran built a successful U.K. based IT company. After twenty-five years at the helm, he sold his business to pursue a greater, more meaningful passion: helping others to find success. Since leaving his company, he has inspired countless people from all walks of life to recognize their strengths and help them hone in on them to find their own paths to success in life and business. He's also expanded his reach by penning multiple books, chapters, and guest posts that spread his proven ideology and methods for individual growth for people of all ages.

Named an Expert Platinum Author, his work has afforded him opportunities to meet and work with people of all ages and learn first-hand what they need to achieve optimal success. One such area that captured his interest is the plight of those living with dementia. Since obtaining a University Diploma on dementia and some considerable research, and following his recent, **"What You Need to Know About Dementia"** , he has now published this book, titled, **"Prevention Of Dementia"** to give hope and clear steps for the prevention of this dreaded disease. It offers insight in an easy-to-digest format that will help anyone who is determined to prevent the onset of Dementia as well as to those who have just been diagnosed with the disease to understand its nuances and know what signs to look for and what questions to ask health care providers.

When not writing or researching, Selva can be found exploring new ways to lift others up and help them live the life of their dreams.

ACKNOWLEDGEMENT

During the last two years of active research into Dementia and while following two University diploma courses on Dementia, my knowledge has been enriched by so many people who have given their time, their research, experiences, opinions and wisdom.

Unfortunately, there is not enough room here to acknowledge each and every one of them. My special heartful thanks go to all those kind people.

Thanks also to my wife Kamini for her support and understanding as I spent long hours while researching and travelling to gather the data required to write this book.

I would also like to thank those who have inspired me, including Pasters T.U. Thomas, Ranjit, Ernest Paul and Rudran.

My heartful thanks also go to those that I couldn't mention. You know who you are!

I cannot end this acknowledgment without giving thanks to God who has provided me with everything I need as illustrated in Philippines 4: Verses 11-13

INTRODUCTION
It is possible to prevent dementia?

As dementia affects millions of people worldwide, the question "if we can prevent it?" arises in everyone's mind. Recent studies show a positive outcome on this matter. According to many studies carried out, there are certainly several ways to prevent or at least delay the onset of dementia. Recognizing the risk factors and working on the modifiable factors can reduce the prevalence.

A study published in the journal *"Lancet Neurology"* *in 2017*, shows possible seven risk factors of dementia. An analysis of data in the population of high-income countries has shown these risk factors to be;

- Physical inactivity
- Smoking
- Midlife hypertension
- Midlife obesity
- Diabetes, depression
- Low educational attainment

This study also suggests applying public health interventions in these areas could substantially prevent the prevalence. *The Lancet commission of dementia prevention, intervention and care* added another two risk factors to the list

- Social isolation
- Midlife hearing loss

This commission then came up with a model that estimates around 35% of dementia cases to be preventable, if dealt with the above risk factors. Hence, preventing dementia is suggested to be possible to a certain extent if interventions are created to build up resilience and healthier lifestyles.

Finnish Geriatric Intervention Study to Prevent Cognitive Impairment and Disability (FINGER) trial that used multimodal interventions such as cognitive training, exercise, diet, and vascular risk monitoring and general health advice showed promising results. The participants were with a low cognitive performance compared to the healthy individuals of their age. The primary outcome of this trial after the 2-year approach was small but beneficial and effective.

At the G8 dementia summit in London on December 2013, the experts noted several facts about prevention and early recognition of dementia. According to this statement by the experts, dementia that is caused mainly due to neurodegenerative diseases e is irreversible. But, modifying risk factors, the strategy involved in preventing cardiovascular diseases, could similarly help in dementia control. Recognizing dementia in its early stages, when the interventions could positively be applied, the progression of dementia could be delayed.

This summit also encourages several lifestyle changes in mid-aged population;

- Smoking cessation

- Exercises – improving physical activeness

- Consuming diets rich in fruit and vegetables and fish (Mediterranean foods)

- Avoiding obesity and diabetes;

- Avoiding excessive alcohol intake;

- Treating high blood pressure.

In other words, they suggest that adopting a healthy lifestyle may help to ward off dementia as it does for other diseases.

In the same manner, the World Dementia Council (WDC) concluded that reducing the risk of dementia to be the only possible way to reduce the number of dementia patients and diseases progression while the world waits for a breakthrough therapy. The council member, Harry John suggests that working on the modifiable risk factors of cardiovascular diseases can positively affect dementia in the same manner. The approach he suggests in his review includes;

- Regular physical activities
- Dealing with diabetes, obesity, smoking and hypertension
- Healthy diet
- Lifelong learning/ cognitive training

According to a statement of evidence of modifiable risk factors of cognitive decline and dementia, the experts suggest that public awareness plays an important role in disease prevention. People should be aware of what science suggests so that they can modify their lifestyle accordingly in order to prevent dementia. Certain healthy behaviours that are known to be effective in preventing and managing diabetes, heart diseases and cancers are proven to positively act on preventing cognitive decline.

With this book, you can understand and deal with the disease, approaching it not with fear, but with confidence. *For More Information, visit:*

www.DementiaPrevention.Care

INDEX

PART II

30 Frequently Asked Questions

CHAPTER 1

The Human Brain & Cognition

The human brain is the main organ that controls the nervous system of a human being. Together with the spinal cord, which is also made up of nerves, it forms the central nervous system. The primary element of the brain, as well as the spinal cord, is nerve cells known as neurons. They are the building blocks that form these large organs and carry out the most complex functions ever found in the world.

The adult human brain weighs about 1.2 – 1.5 kg, which is around 2% of the body weight. This organ controls many functions of the body starting from signalling every possible activity we do, to the maintenance of the body's chemical balance. One of the most complex human brain functions is the cognition. While many scientists struggle for decades to identify exactly how these complex functions are carried out by the brain, the complete knowledge is not yet achieved.

What is cognition? Cognition is how a human understands the world and act accordingly. It is a group of mental abilities and processes that take part in nearly every human action. Cognitive abilities are brain-controlled skills that are necessary for a human to carry out any task of any degree (simple – complex). Further, these abilities have a lot to do with learning, remembering, problem-solving and paying attention. As an example, a simple action as if receiving a call represents a major role of cognition; perception is required to answer the phone (hearing the ringtone), decision making to decide if answering or not, motor skills are needed to lift the receiver, language skills are necessary to communicate over the phone and social skills are needed to interpret the tone of voice and to interact properly with another human being.

There are specific neuron networks that control different cognitive functions and are located in different areas of the brain. As an example, memory skills rely mainly on frontal and the temporal lobes of the brain as the neuron network that works on creating new memories are located in these areas. Likewise, there are certain areas of the brain that controls perception, memory recall, logical thinking, concentration and other skills.

Cognitive functions of the brain

There are several cognitive functions of the brain and they are involved in a set of different skills.

Cognitive function	Skills involved
Perception	Recognition of senses and their interpretation (Smell, touch, hearing, special details, etc.)
Attention	Ability to continue concentrating on a particular object, action, or thought. Also the ability to overcome the disturbances from the environment.
Memory	Short-term memory (limited storage) Long-term memory (unlimited storage)

Motor functions	Ability to mobilize the muscles of the body and manipulate any object.
Language and comprehension	Skills to recognize and translate sounds heard into words and to create a verbal output. This also includes the ability to create words in order to create understandable sentences and skills to describe an event, object or a person in an understandable way.
Visual and spatial processing	Ability to process the visual details, to understand the spatial relationship of the objects. The skills also

	involve in recognizing images and scenarios.
Executive functions	Skills that enable goal-oriented behaviour, as of the ability to plan, and execute a goal. These include: **Flexibility** – the ability to quickly switch to the appropriate mental mode to carry out a certain function. **Theory of mind** – Understanding other people's inner world, their needs, intentions, their likes and dislikes.

	Anticipation – making predictions by recognizing patterns.
	Problem-solving – recognizing a problem in the right way and then create solutions accordingly.
	Decision making – the ability to make decisions assisted with other cognitive skills.
	Working Memory – the capacity to receive and manipulate information in real time.
	Emotional self-regulation - the ability to express, identify and

<table>
<tr><td></td><td>

manage one's own emotions.

Sequencing – the ability of a person to break down complex actions or tasks into manageable smaller units and organize them in the right order.

Inhibition – the ability to resist distraction, and internal urges.

</td></tr>
</table>

All these cognitive functions listed above are controlled completely by the brain. While they are optimum in a healthy young individual, there is a common cognitive decline recognized in many elderly individuals. Anyhow, cognitive decline is not a normal part of ageing although ageing can increase the probability of it.

Certain brain diseases, lifestyle factors and health states can increase the inefficiency of the neuron networks that carry out cognitive functions and it is when a condition known as "dementia" is recognized. The minor cognitive decline due to ageing might not progress to severe stages, but dementia progresses in most of the cases and applies a huge burden to the national health care services and costs. That is why it is necessary to understand the brain, its functions, and risk factors of developing dementia and to work in the aim of reducing the prevalence of dementia and related cognitive decline.

CHAPTER 2

Dementia

The human brain is made up of millions of nerve cells, and like any other cells in the body, these cells are susceptible to "wear and tear". If the nerve cells of the brain degenerate or damage, the memory and the other cognitive functions can get disturbed. There are many reasons that lead to cognitive dysfunctions, and one of the most common reasons has been recognized as degenerative changes of the ageing brain. Human ageing does not affect only the skin and the appearance of a person but also affects all the cells of the body including nerve cells. Dementia is not a part of normal ageing although growing old increases the risk of dementia.

The loss of memory, thinking and reasoning are altogether known as "dementia". As this condition progresses, many people would show related behavioural changes that interfere with their daily activities and life. The cognitive brain controls many important human functions such as memory, comprehension, visual perception, logical thinking, self-management, focus and concentration. Therefore, people who suffer from dementia will show changes in the above-mentioned abilities.

Dementia is also known as "major neurocognitive disorder" even though it is not a disease itself. It is an umbrella term used to signify a range of symptoms. The degree of severity of this condition may vary from mild to severe. Though at the beginning a person might only show signs of memory disturbances, as the disease progresses he might completely depend on another person even for their basic activities of life.

<u>Causes of Dementia</u>

Various factors and conditions contribute to the development of dementia. Starting from degenerative conditions of the brain cells to the use of alcohol and drugs, there are several factors recognized to increase the risk of loss of memory and other cognitive functions. The most frequent causes of dementia or dementia-like conditions include:

- Degenerative neurological disorders: Alzheimer's disease, Parkinson's disease, Huntington's disease and multiple sclerosis. In these conditions, the symptoms get worse over time.

- Vascular disorders: Conditions that may interfere with the blood circulation of the brain can also cause cognitive dysfunctions.

- Trauma: Injuries to the brain can damage the nerve cells in the centres that control functions such as memory, comprehension, thinking, focus and concentration. Road traffic accidents, falls from height and even concussions can affect these centres of the brain, resulting in dementia.

- Infections of the brain: Infectious diseases such as meningitis, encephalitis, HIV and Creutzfeldt-Jakob disease can cause dementia. Most of these conditions can be improved by treating the infectious process.

- Long terms use of alcohol and drugs

- Hydrocephalus – a fluid buildup of the brain.

Neurodegenerative diseases and dementia

Neurodegenerative diseases are the conditions that cause progressive degeneration or death of nerve cells. These conditions are incurable, irreversible and debilitating. The human brain and the spinal cord are made up of the neurons and when they get damaged or die, they cannot be replaced. Therefore, conditions that cause degenerative changes in the brain cells cannot be treated and progresses over time. If a person suffers from dementia due to neurodegenerative conditions, their symptoms of loss of memory, concentration, focus, thought process progress as time passes by. In the most advanced cases, behavioural changes, self-care and even communication will be greatly affected.

Dementia is the main concern of most of the degenerative brain diseases, and they are;

- Alzheimer's disease (AD)
- Parkinson's disease (PD) and PD-related disorders
- Prion disease
- Motor neurone diseases (MND)
- Huntington's disease (HD)
- Spinocerebellar ataxia (SCA)
- Spinal muscular atrophy (SMA)

Out of all conditions listed above 60-70% of dementia is a result of Alzheimer's disease.

Neurodegenerative diseases are linked with age and that is why an ageing population carries a higher risk of dementia.

Vascular Dementia

Vascular dementia is the next most common reason for dementia after Alzheimer's disease. It is a result of conditions that interfere with the blood circulation of the brain. Conditions such as high cholesterol levels, stroke, uncontrolled high blood pressure and brain bleeds are responsible for cognitive decline. As in neurodegenerative disorders, ageing increases the risk of vascular dementia. In addition, advanced heart diseases can also increase the risk of this type of dementia.

Symptoms in vascular dementia can appear gradually or rapidly, depending on the underlying condition. Confusion, misunderstanding and loss of memory are common early signs. As the condition progresses, people struggle to finish chores with limited attention spans. Visual disturbances and hallucinations might also manifest in this condition.

<u>Alcohol-Related Brain Damage (ARBD)</u>

Alcohol-related brain damage takes place when a person regularly drinking too much alcohol over several years. ARBD includes several conditions such as Wernicke-Korsakoff syndrome and alcoholic dementia. None of these conditions causes irreversibly progressive loss of memory and cognition. In contrast to neurodegenerative conditions, people with ARBD can partially or fully recover by remaining alcohol-free and receiving good support.

ARBD is a result of excessive consumption of alcohol and related deficiency of Vitamin B1 (thiamine). While alcohol is toxic for the human cells, vitamin B1 is necessary to produce energy within the cells. Brain cells are the human cells that use the most amount of energy.

Constant consumption of excessive alcohol causes a toxic damage to the cells while causing vitamin B1 deficiency. This toxicity can create a chemical change in the brain and interfere with its functions. Also, heavy drinking is linked with poor diet and damage of stomach lining which can cause vitamin B1 deficiency. Therefore, the brain cells of the heavy drinkers deprive of energy and are showered with toxins that can damage or reduce the efficacy of the functions of the brain cells.

Alcohol can further cause repeated head injuries due to frequent falls and getting into fights.

What does excessive alcohol consumption mean? For men, it could mean consuming more than 50 units of alcohol per week, and for women, more than 35 units per week. Consuming such high levels of alcohol also lead to alcohol addiction and over several years it can damage the brain, causing alcohol-related brain damage (ARBD) in some people.

Types of Dementia

Dementia can be divided into two groups according to the involvement of different parts of the brain

Cortical dementia

Cortical dementia is defined as dementia due to the problems involving the cerebral cortex, the outer part of the brain. The areas of brain cortex play an essential role in memory and language. People who suffer from cortical dementia manifest a higher degree of symptoms such as severe memory loss and severe problems with comprehension and understanding. Alzheimer's disease and Creutzfeldt-Jakob disease are recognized as causing cortical dementia.

Subcortical dementia

Subcortical dementia occurs due to problems of the parts of the brain beneath the brain cortex. Individuals affected with this type of dementia manifest changes in the speed of thinking and ability to initiate activities. Memory loss and comprehension problems involve to a lesser degree. Parkinson's disease, Huntington's disease and HIV cause subcortical dementia.

Certain types of dementia involve both parts of the brain, and their symptoms can manifest a mix of cortical as well as subcortical dementia.

Some professionals also classify dementia into five main categories;

Alzheimer's disease	This is the most common form of dementia. According to records, about over five million Alzheimer's patients were present in 2015 in the USA. Further, the records demonstrate that a new person start showing symptoms of this condition every sixty-seven seconds. As the chemistry of the brain changes, bewilderment and unusual temperament variations are noticed in these individuals with Alzheimer's disease.

Vascular dementia	The second most common type of dementia and is due to problems with the blood circulation and vascular diseases of the brain and body.
Lewy body dementia	Lewy Body Dementia is rare and is distinguished by sleep disturbances, memory loss, slowed gait, hallucinations and problems with body balancing. There are currently 1.3 million patients who suffer from Lewy body dementia in the US. Protein deposits that are known as Lewy bodies deposit in the nerve cells disturbing the chemical signal conduction in the brain.

Frontotemporal dementia	This is the fourth most common type of dementia and is characterized by changes in personality and behaviour, language problems and comprehension (using gestures in place of words, and incomplete or vague sentences). The cause of this condition is yet unknown and believed to link with a genetic mutation. Frontotemporal Dementia involves frontal and sides regions of the brain.
Additional forms of dementia	Includes all the types of dementia not listed in the above four categories and mixed dementia. Mixed dementia is when two types of dementia manifest together in a single person.

Stages of Dementia

Dementia is progressive most of the time when caused due to neurodegenerative diseases, vascular diseases or Lewy body formation. The progression of this condition can be divided into three stages; early stage, middle stage and late stage.

Early stage of dementia

The early stage of dementia will show mild symptoms such as simple forgetfulness. Incidents such as forgetting the chequebook at home, forgetting someone's name or walking to the room and forgetting why he went there are commonly described by many patients at this stage. Yes, these can also be signs of the normal ageing process as many individuals are a little forgetful after 65 years of age. Anyhow, the signs of dementia at this stage seem all normal and need a professional consultation to see if this is a progressive condition.

This stage of dementia does not interfere with an individual's daily living. These patients can live and function independently, even though support from friends and family could be of great help.

Middle stage of dementia

Even at this stage, individuals will not show severe dysfunctions of a wide array of cognitive functions. The patients can still function individually, but, would require more attention and care from a caregiver or friends and family.

At this stage individuals would need assistance in managing finances, dressing up and bathing as they frequently experience confusion and memory loss. There might also be noticeable sleep pattern changes such as sleeping during the day and restlessness at night that needs to be dealt with.

<u>Late stage of dementia</u>

At this stage, brain damage is extensive and is marked by behaviours that are out of the individual's character. These include increased agitation, continual questioning, pacing, and unusual sleep patterns. Late-stage dementia can be further characterized by physical symptoms such as muscle weakness, weight loss, appetite suppression, inability to swallow and inability to walk, sit up, or hold their head up. The control of defecation and urination will also be affected and care should be provided for these individuals all the time. These individuals cannot function independently and as this stage progresses individuals may become bed-ridden.

<u>Signs & Symptoms</u>

Dementia affects the cognitive sphere of the brain at first. But, in later stages, the symptoms can include comprehension difficulties, problems with visual and spatial perception, behavioural and psychological changes and physical signs and symptoms.

Cognitive symptoms

Simple memory loss is the foremost common sign of dementia. Professionals believe that there can be a difference in memory loss due to ageing and dementia. It is believed that forgetting names and things of the people whom they meet rarely are a sign of ageing, while forgetting names and things of the dear ones and of whom they meet frequently are a sign of dementia. The short-term memory disturbances in dementia include, confusion, problems recalling recent events, struggles in creating new memories and difficulty in concentration and organization. Even simple steps of preparing a meal can be a huge struggle for these individuals. Difficulty in making decisions and problem-solving can be challenging too.

Comprehension and language challenges

These signs and symptoms develop in advanced stages and include difficulty in recalling a conversation, aphasia or difficulty to recall the correct words to identify something and early evening confusion (also known as sundowning).

Visual and spatial skills

These skills are further affected as dementia progresses. Difficulty in estimating the distance, perceiving objects in its dimensions and confusion about the location, date and time can frequently be observed. Therefore, individuals might find it difficult to climb or descend stairs, recognize objects and recall where they locate. It is necessary to take care of these individuals and keep under observation as if they go outside alone they may not remember their way to come back home.

Behavioural and psychological symptoms

The late stage of dementia includes behavioural changes. Temperament changes, lack of self-control, agitation, or roaming and becoming lost are a few common signs. Many individuals have a social withdrawal and would isolate themselves.

Depression, delusion, hallucination and paranoia may accompany as well.

Physical symptoms

Many physical functions can get affected by dementia; body balance, hand grip, time needed to stand from a seated position, gait with shorter or unsteady steps, gait with one side weaker than the other, numbness in extremities, physical weakness, inability to combine muscle movements, and jumbled speech are all physical signs accompany with dementia.

Dementia Facts and Figures

Worldwide

According to the World Health Organization (WHO), around 50 million people suffer from dementia around the world. 60% out of these individuals are from low- to middle- income countries. The estimated general population aged 60 and over with dementia at a given time is between 5 to 8 per every 100 people. Therefore, an increasing ageing population further increases the risk of dementia in future years.

Every year WHO records more than 10 million new cases of dementia from around the world. This means one new person develops dementia every 3 seconds. In 2030, the number of people who suffer from dementia is estimated to rise up to 82 million and in 2050 up to 152 million. Majority of these individuals are expected to be from the developing countries of the world.

Dementia costs a lot for the world economy. In 2015 it cost the world around $818 billion and it is estimated to rise up to 2 trillion by 2030.

<u>USA</u>

Alzheimer's disease is the 6th leading cause of death in the US. 1 in 3 seniors die from Alzheimer's or another type of dementia and it kills more than breast cancer and prostate cancer combined. 16.1 million Americans provide unpaid care for people with dementia and it costs over $232 billion for the country. Early diagnosis is estimated to save up to $ 7.9 trillion in medical care. Every 65 seconds a new person develops dementia and it is estimated that by the year of 2050 5.7 million Americans will suffer from this condition. The United States alone estimate a rise of the cost up to $ 1.1 trillion by 2050.

UK

The United Kingdom also shows a similarly high prevalence of dementia. It is estimated that 850,000 individuals live with dementia in the UK at the moment, but only 537,097 individuals are diagnosed. Statistics predict that the number of individuals with dementia will rise up to 2 million by 2050. In the UK dementia is the only condition in the top 10 causes of death without a treatment to cure or reduce the progression.

Dementia costs £ 26 billion in the UK. The majority of the cost is due to informal, social and medical care. The statistics show if dementia could be delayed by five years, it could save up to £ 21.2 billion every year by 2050.

The global movement of dementia prevention and management

World Health Organization (WHO) has developed seven action areas and targets to tackle the rising concern of dementia, increasing prevalence and rising costs.

1. **Dementia to be managed as a public health priority**

   This involves the development of national policies, strategies, plans and frameworks for prevention, early diagnosis and effective management of dementia and its symptoms. This will involve 75% of countries worldwide by 2025.

2. **Dementia awareness and creating a friendly environment**

   By 2025, 100% of countries worldwide will have functional ongoing public-awareness campaigns on dementia. By 2025 50% of countries will have a minimum of 1-2 dementia friendly initiatives.

3. Dementia risk reduction

A global action plan is created and carried out worldwide.

4. Dementia diagnosis and care

WHO works together with countries to diagnose a minimum 50% dementia cases in 50% of countries in the world by 2025.

5. Care and support for dementia patients

By 2025 75% of the countries will be able to provide enough support and training for the caregivers and family who look after dementia patients.

6. Information system for dementia

By 2025 50% of countries will be able to collect data of key indicators of dementia. This will further help in future action plans and prevention strategies in the coming years.

7. Dementia research and innovation

Global research output on dementia is estimated to double before 2025.

CHAPTER 3

Is It Possible To Prevent Dementia?

As dementia affects millions of people worldwide, the question "if we can prevent it?" arises in everyone's mind. Recent studies show a positive outcome on this matter. According to many studies carried out, there are certainly several ways to prevent or at least delay the onset of dementia. Recognizing the risk factors and working on the modifiable factors can reduce the prevalence.

A study published in the journal *"Lancet Neurology"* *in 2017,* shows possible seven risk factors of dementia. An analysis of data in the population of high-income countries has shown these risk factors to be;

- Physical inactivity
- Smoking
- Midlife hypertension
- Midlife obesity
- Diabetes, depression
- Low educational attainment

This study also suggests applying public health interventions in these areas could substantially prevent the prevalence. *The Lancet commission of dementia prevention, intervention and care* added another two risk factors to the list

- Social isolation
- Midlife hearing loss

This commission then came up with a model that estimates around 35% of dementia cases to be preventable, if dealt with the above risk factors. Hence, preventing dementia is suggested to be possible to a certain extent if interventions are created to build up resilience and healthier lifestyles.

Finnish Geriatric Intervention Study to Prevent Cognitive Impairment and Disability (FINGER) trial that used multimodal interventions such as cognitive training, exercise, diet, and vascular risk monitoring and general health advice showed promising results. The participants were with a low cognitive performance compared to the healthy individuals of their age. The primary outcome of this trial after the 2-year approach was small but beneficial and effective.

At the G8 dementia summit in London on December 2013, the experts noted several facts about prevention and early recognition of dementia. According to this statement by the experts, dementia that is caused mainly due to neurodegenerative diseases e is irreversible. But, modifying risk factors, the strategy involved in preventing cardiovascular diseases, could similarly help in dementia control. Recognizing dementia in its early stages, when the interventions could positively be applied, the progression of dementia could be delayed.

This summit also encourages several lifestyle changes in mid-aged population;

- Smoking cessation
- Exercises – improving physical activeness
- Consuming diets rich in fruit and vegetables and fish (Mediterranean foods)
- Avoiding obesity and diabetes;
- Avoiding excessive alcohol intake;
- Treating high blood pressure.

In other words, they suggest that adopting a healthy lifestyle may help to ward off dementia as it does for other diseases.

In the same manner, the World Dementia Council (WDC) concluded that reducing the risk of dementia to be the only possible way to reduce the number of dementia patients and diseases progression while the world waits for a breakthrough therapy. The council member, Harry John suggests that working on the modifiable risk factors of cardiovascular diseases can positively affect dementia in the same manner. The approach he suggests in his review includes;

- Regular physical activities
- Dealing with diabetes, obesity, smoking and hypertension
- Healthy diet
- Lifelong learning/ cognitive training

According to a statement of evidence of modifiable risk factors of cognitive decline and dementia, the experts suggest that public awareness plays an important role in disease prevention. People should be aware of what science suggests so that they can modify their lifestyle accordingly in order to prevent dementia. Certain healthy behaviours that are known to be effective in preventing and managing diabetes, heart diseases and cancers are proven to positively act on preventing cognitive decline.

CHAPTER 4

Risk Factors that Matter

There are several risk factors for cognitive decline and dementia. Many of these risk factors are modifiable and by dealing with them, it is possible to delay the onset or slow the progression of this condition. Some people may have memory problems due to lack of vitamins such as vitamin B12 which is essential for healthy brain cells. A gland in the neck called "thyroid gland" release "thyroxin" which is an important hormone for the body. A reduction in this hormone can be a reversible risk factor for dementia. Moreover, some infectious diseases can also increase the risk of having memory problems. Fortunately, these risks are completely modifiable, and memory difficulties will regularly improve and resolve.

Alzheimer's disease

More than 2/3 of patients of dementia are due to Alzheimer's disease. The exact causes of this condition aren't clearly known until now but there are some theories that suggest reasons such as genetic factors, ageing and neurodegeneration. Alzheimer disease may be common in some families with an early onset due to gene mutations. These mutations may disrupt the natural balance of protein content in brain tissues causing significant deterioration of brain functions.

Another common risk for this health problem is ageing since people more than 65 years old are at higher risk of dementia and this risk even increases more as a person gets older.

Some researchers also suggest that daily exposure to aluminium such as by the use of cooking foils and cans is associated with dementia. However, this area is still under study and no confirmation reached yet.

<u>Diabetes Type 2</u>

Type 2 diabetes hits individuals usually in the late thirties. This condition carries a serious risk of developing cognitive problems and dementia. Recent studies proved that diabetic patients are more prone to dementia compared to their peers who have normal blood glucose levels. Even people who don't have diabetes but suffer from insulin resistance or decreased insulin release may be at risk of suffering from dementia. It was also found that diabetic patients who are receiving antidiabetic drugs have a lower incidence of cognitive decline in contrast to untreated patients.

The way diabetes may impair cognitive abilities and memory is explained as high glucose level in the blood causing harmful effects on the brain cells. When glucose level increases in blood, insulin should play its role to trap this sugar to be stored in liver cells. However, people who have type 2 diabetes can't perform this step as they have decreased insulin secretion and lower insulin sensitivity. Excess blood glucose will be directed to other pathways producing toxic substances that may harm brain cells affecting their power and functions. The more a patient has uncontrolled diabetes, the higher the negative impact on brain cells increasing the chance to have dementia and impaired cognition. Uncontrolled diabetes can also cause several problems on blood vessels including brain blood circulation. These problems vary from clot formations, thickening, and weakening of blood vessels leading to an inadequate blood supply to brain cells and raise the risk of dementia.

High cholesterol

A high cholesterol profile is more likely to promote a condition called "atherosclerosis". It is the thickening of blood vessels walls due to continuous deposition of excessive cholesterol. This can impair the quality of blood circulation as it increases the affinity of blood vessels walls to form blood clots which will narrow the lumen and affect the blood flow to the brain. Subsequently, brain cells may not have adequate nutrition and proper circulation to get rid of wastes and by the time their function begins to deteriorate and thus, may affect memory and learning abilities. Diabetic patients also have more liability to encounter this problem as their bodies are more susceptible to form blood clots on top of the thick blood vessels walls.

<u>Depression</u>

There is a close relationship between depression and dementia. Depression may be a symptom of dementia, and sometimes depressive behaviours such as lack of concentration and detachment can look like dementia. Depressed patients usually keep themselves away from social interactions which may contribute to dementia. This loneliness, particularly in older ages is extremely harmful to mental health. Some studies showed that the risk of dementia is almost two times more in depressed patients than in the others. This risk rises more when patients suffer from high blood pressure accompanied by depression as both together may trigger strokes and impaired brain circulation. Psychiatrists always encourage these patients to socialize more often and attend sessions of group therapy to improve their conditions and avoid progressive cognitive decline and dementia.

Sleep problems

For a healthy brain and body, good sleep is required to ensure that both are working well. Poor sleep, especially in patients who suffer from frequent waking up at night, may be detrimental to brain functions. Many researchers discussed this topic focusing more in a condition called "sleep apnea" which is a breathing disorder that prevents continuous night sleep and makes patients wake up several times as they cease breathing several times during sleep. This problem is more serious in older patient and can harm the cognitive abilities of patients in this age.

Furthermore, since sleep is required to help brain cells excrete unwanted toxins and lethal proteins, lack of adequate night sleep can cause over accumulation of these substances in brain cells affecting their functionality. As time passes, these toxins may even cause cell damage and a significant decline in cognitive power and memory.

Head injury

Head trauma is another serious condition that may harm brain cognition. About 2 % of US citizens have long-term memory problems such as dementia due to brain trauma and this percentage is even more in other countries. Injuries to the brain are more harmful in older people as they increase the incidence of developing dementia. A study in JAMA Neurology showed that brain trauma markedly increased the risk of dementia in people older than 55 years old, while less severe brain injuries caused more liability to dementia in 56 and more age group. Early exposure to head injury was also found to be associated with a higher incidence of dementia at older ages. Moreover, head trauma is believed to be the most common environmental risk factor for cognitive decline and memory disabilities. This risk may vary depending on personal and social variations. For example, highly educated people with higher IQ may encounter less brain impairment. In addition, lifestyle, career success and social activities are all factors that may decrease the effect of brain injury in cognitive functions.

Smoking

Smoking cigarette markedly increases the risk of mental deterioration and developing dementia. This was proved by multiple studies that highlighted the role of smoking in worsening the quality of blood vessels which impair blood circulation to the brain and make patients more liable to cognitive disorders.

Furthermore, cigarettes contain several toxic substances and chemicals that may cause direct damage to brain tissues. The exact mechanism of this is still unclear and there are even some theories suggesting that the "nicotine" in cigarettes may decrease the risk of dementia.

Some researchers also stated that smoking can increase the risk of dementia by around one third compared to non-smokers. The risk of having dementia increases depending on the number of daily smoked cigarettes. However, quitting smoking as early as possible can gradually decrease this incidence.

Alcohol intake

Drinking alcohol may be associated with dementia. According to the amount of daily alcohol intake, the incidence of mental decline may increase. Usually drinking mild to moderate amount of alcohol is not associated with high risk of dementia. Some studies even found that this light consumption may have a protective effect on the brain. Moreover, studies on people who are suffering from dementia found that alcohol intake in these patients is associated with more brain deterioration.

Moderate consumption of alcohol can increase the concentration of good cholesterol, decrease risks of heart diseases, improve brain circulation and decrease inflammation. However, consuming large quantities of alcohol and frequent binge drinking are detrimental to brain cells and may also predispose to strokes.

Dementia associated with great alcohol consumption is called Alcohol-Related Brain Damage (ARBD) which is highly linked with middle-aged individuals. It is believed that alcohol has more influence on females than males due to hormonal causes. However, more cases of men are diagnosed with alcohol-related brain damage possibly as men tend to drink alcohol more than women.

Another condition of dementia related to alcohol consumption is a disease called "Wernicke Korsakoff syndrome". This problem can be hardly diagnosed during the lifetime and more likely to be discovered after death. The reason for this illness is that alcohol consumers have inadequate absorption of vitamin B1. Consequently, the deficiency of this essential vitamin decreases brain cognitive abilities and cause memory impairment. This condition is characterized by difficulties in learning new things, and great gaps in long-term memory.

<u>Heart and vessels diseases</u>

Health problems related to heart and blood vessels contribute to brain deterioration and dementia. The reason for this may be that heart diseases such as heart attack and rhythm irregularities can be serious risks for more vascular events including vessels that supply the brain. A new study found that elderly women with heart disorders are more likely to suffer from signs and symptoms of dementia in their advanced ages.

High blood pressure can also add more danger as it gradually harms the quality of blood circulation and causes other serious problems. Therefore, cardiologists advise cardiac patients to keep their blood pressure controlled, do regular exercises, and eat healthy food to enhance body and brain circulation and prevent brain decline.

Gender

The incidence of Alzheimer's diseases related dementia is higher in women when compared to men. This may be due to the fact that the average lifetime of women is more than the men, so they are more likely to suffer from symptoms of impaired brain functions. Furthermore, some theories link between the hormonal deficiency that occurs after menopause and impaired mental functions. These theories also found that hormone replacement therapy in women after menopause may reduce the risk of Alzheimer's related dementia. Hormone replacement therapy administered after menopause also shows to improve other symptoms related to this period of life. However, it is not recommended to use this treatment only to decrease the danger of dementia.

Women and men have an equal risk of developing other types of dementia. Men have a higher risk of vascular dementia as the incidence of heart diseases and stroke are more in males.

Ageing

It is considered the most established risk factor for dementia. People after the age of 65 are more prone to suffer from cognitive decline although there is a small incidence of dementia at earlier ages. This effect is thought to be due to other health problems associated with the ageing process such as high blood pressure, defects in the natural ability of the body to repair cell damage, sex hormones deficiency, weaker immune system, and increased danger of heart diseases and strokes.

All of these factors do not only affect brain cells but have a wide influence on all body cells in decreasing their power and quality of natural physiological processes. As people age, functions of the brain cells may be affected due to disruption of brain circulation and increased toxic pressure on the cells as a result of senility.

Ethnicity

It is believed that some communities are more likely to develop dementia than others. For instance, south Asian citizens may have a higher incidence of dementia particularly of vascular type due to increased risk of heart diseases and strokes. Furthermore, African communities also seem to have a higher incidence of dementia. The cause of this may be the lifestyle, dietary habits, and smoking which increase the danger of diabetes and stroke.

<u>Genetics</u>

The Genetic role in developing dementia is still unclear. However, it was seen that dementia may be inherited in some families. Some studies found that around 20 genes may affect the risk of developing dementia. For example, having a parent with Alzheimer's diseases may increase the chance of having the same condition in contrast to other people. Furthermore, in rare conditions inheriting genes that can directly be a reason for dementia may occur. Some families may have familial Alzheimer's disease that passes from one generation to others.

CHAPTER 5

Risk Factors Reduction

The risk of having dementia can be reduced by adopting several habits and by taking some precautions. Starting a healthy lifestyle with a balanced diet and regular physical activities can contribute to a higher quality of brain functions and decrease the ability to suffer from brain decline. The earlier an individual begins these lifestyle changes, the better the result in the long run. However, it is nevver too late to start changing unhealthy habits that may increase the risk of dementia.

Dementia can be prevented by lowering the incidence of other diseases that may contribute to dementia such as diabetes, high blood pressure, and heart diseases, in addition to dietary modifications, smoking cessation, and treatment of psychological disturbances such as depression.

Mental activities

Dementia can be described as the process of shrinkage of the brain while getting older. This process is a part of ageing that happens to older people particularly after 65 years of age. Thinkers, writers, readers, musicians, multi-tongue speaker are some examples of people who may use their mind frequently have a lower risk and late onset of symptoms.

Generally, frequent usage of brain functions is an important preventive measure to decrease the risk of dementia. Mental activities such as reading, playing games that stimulate mental abilities, learning different languages, playing music are all things that may improve brain power and delay the symptoms of dementia.

"Use it or lose it" is a general statement that can be applied in this situation. Involvement of brain cells in several activities like these can decrease the cognitive deterioration that happens while ageing as it helps brain cells to build more nerve connection between each other. This nerve connection is called "neuron density" and is essential to maintain the quality of cognitive functions.

Some specific brain games such as playing cards and board games play a key role in activating concentration and enhancing memory. A regular playing of such games in younger ages may lower the risk of having dementia after the age of 65.

People who are employed in jobs that require higher mental activities are also less likely to develop cognitive decline after retirement. These jobs include musicians, civil engineers, and architects. It was found that workers in such jobs that involve working with high complexity data have higher cognitive abilities and seem to be at lower risk of developing dementia.

Brain training is a term that describes exercising brain cells. it is a way to prevent developing cognitive decline at old age and can improve the level of intelligence as well. Many scientists studied this area and found that brain training activities can be crucial to brain health. It may enhance brain plasticity, which is the ability of brain cells to adapt to new changes and learn new things. Brain training help in maintaining a higher IQ level even later in life. This alone can be a strong guard against symptoms of dementia such as memory loss and cognitive disabilities.

A good example of brain training is to be committed to rewarding tasks that need high brain power such as reading, writing, or learning a new language. Regular performance of such activities exercises the brain's abilities challenge brain cells to maximize their perfection.

<u>Physical activity</u>

Vascular dementia is the second most common type of dementia after Alzheimer's disease. This typically occurs due to vascular events such as strokes that impair brain blood circulation and affect brain functions. By increasing the level of physical activities, it is possible to lower the risk of developing heart diseases, diabetes, and high blood pressure which are common reasons for strokes. Moreover, physical exercises improve the level of body cholesterol, help weight reduction and contribute to psychological balance which altogether can reduce the risk of cognitive decline. In general, a sedentary lifestyle is harmful to all body tissues including brain cells. So, it is always advised to perform more physical activities to improve blood circulation and avoid the accumulation of toxic substances and wastes of biological processes. A study examined the relationship between sedentary lifestyle and cognitive decline in normal people who don't have dementia. The results showed that physical activities have a remarkable guarding role against cognitive deterioration. Furthermore, physical activities were seen also to reduce the progression of dementia in Alzheimer's disease.

Any type of physical activity can contribute to the cognitive ability of the brain starting from slight walking to vigorous muscular exercises.

Apart from the influence of exercise on preventing vascular dementia, it can also stimulate the formation of new neuron connections in the brain. In addition, physical activities can trigger the release of protective proteins that improve the quality and survival of nerve cells.

To accomplish these effects, it is recommended to have regular 30 minutes exercises 3-5 times weekly that allow increasing heart rate and induce sweating. Brisk walking, cycling, and swimming on a regular basis can be enough to gain their beneficial effects of reducing the risk of dementia.

<u>Stop smoking</u>

It is advised to stop smoking as early as possible due to its harmful effects on brain power and cognitive abilities. Stopping smoking at any time of life may participate in decreasing the risk of dementia. Surely, the earlier smoking is stopped, the less the risk to suffer from brain deterioration will be. But, as said before it is never too late to quit smoking as there will be always a benefit from this on brain health. Since smoking may increase the risk of heart diseases, disrupt cholesterol profile, and rise liability to strokes, stopping it can be a vital decision to avoid detrimental effects on brain health including dementia.

After cessation of smoking, blood pressure and heart rate start to return to normal and the concentration of blood oxygen rises gradually to its normal range. With time, toxic substances of smoking will be eliminated from blood which improves blood circulation and facilitates a higher level of brain functioning.

Socializing

An involvement in social activities can bring out multiple beneficial impacts on brain and body health. Scientists found that being socially active lower the risk of developing brain decline and Alzheimer's disease. The reason for this may be related to the role of social events in engaging the brain while sharing information and may also include involvement in group physical activities like playing games and teamwork. The idea of sharing thoughts and learning from others while socializing greatly contribute to the quality of brain cells and enhance new nerve connections formation. Socializing as well is a good protector against depression and other psychological problems that may be a part of dementia.

Lose weight

Having a healthy weight can protect the body from several health problems such as diabetes, heart diseases and high blood pressure. All of these problems are common risk factors for developing dementia in older ages of life. So, monitoring body weight and avoiding excessive accumulation of fats can reduce the risk of brain decline symptoms. Dieticians recommend eating a balanced diet rich in minerals and vitamins, with low calories and fats to be in shape. Exercise also is essential as it helps burn excess fats and calories.

Being overweight in midlife can be closely associated with dementia due to Alzheimer's diseases and vascular events. Thus, controlling weight in this period of life is an essential preventive measure of dementia.

Avoid excessive alcohol intake

Since consuming large amounts of alcohol is known to be a serious risk for dementia, it is advised for alcohol drinkers to decrease their alcohol intake. According to NHS, the recommended level of alcohol consumption is not to exceed 14 units weekly for both sexes and should be consumed over more than three days. This amount can be measured as about five glasses of wine each week. Anyhow, it can be a great choice to stop drinking alcohol gradually to experience better mental abilities. This can be achieved gradually by drinking smaller glasses every time and alternate between soft and hard drinks.

Good sleep

In general, Sleeping well contributes to a healthier brain and body. One precious benefit of having enough sleep of around 7-8 hours every night is the reduction of Alzheimer's disease. Good sleep quality helps brain cells to avoid the accumulation of unwanted proteins that can gradually affect brain cognitive functions. Moreover, excess sleep more than nine hours daily can be also associated with higher liability to develop dementia.

Avoid psychiatric disorders

Depression is closely associated with dementia. It is considered as risk factor for brain decline and a symptom of dementia as well. Suffering from depressive symptoms particularly in mid-life was found to be a serious risk factor for developing dementia after the age of 65 years. Thus, it is wise to avoid depression and start a treatment plan as early as possible to decrease the chance of experiencing declined brain functions.

Depression itself has several forms of severity and there are some warning symptoms that should be monitored to avoid suffering from severe depression. It is advised to prevent depression rather than treating it, which all contribute to decreasing detrimental effects on brain health.

Psychiatrists recommend keeping eyes on signs such as social withdrawal, isolation, difficulties in concentration, and continuous anxiety as alarms towards more serious mental disorders. Treating depression in patients of Alzheimer's disease may involve social therapies and medications. The aim of treatment is to try to add pleasure and hope to the mind of the patient. All of this can be reflected on both depression symptoms and in improved cognitive abilities.

Nervous personalities seem to have a higher risk of Alzheimer's dementia. Nervousness may be associated with a higher risk of stress and pressure. In contrast, calm personalities may be at lower risk of dementia. It is generally advised to avoid stressful events and minimize the level of anxiety by performing relaxing activities regularly to chill out. Doing this routinely will give the chance for the brain cells to relax and recover.

<u>Nutrition</u>

As mentioned earlier, overweight can increase the chance of having dementia in old age due to several reasons. Losing weight is a challenging task which requires a strict schedule of both diet plans and physical activities. Replacing unhealthy food with healthier options is a good step towards delaying symptoms of dementia.

In the next chapter, there will be more details about how dietary modifications can decrease the risk of dementia.

In general, reducing consumption of alcoholic beverages may have a protective role, eating more green vegetables and fresh fruits have an additional antioxidant effect which guards the brain cells against ageing and oxidative damage.

Omega-3 which is found in oily fish such as salmon may also play a protective role due to its high nutritional value. It is always recommended by the dieticians to feed young infants with a diet rich in omega-3 to enhance their brain development. Based on the same idea, omega-3 can be beneficial for adults to prevent cognitive decline as they get older. However, a confirmed effect of omega-3 on reducing the risk of dementia is still not confirmed.

Red and white meats may increase the risk of dementia as they have a higher concentration of saturated fats. On the other hand, fish is more helpful for brain cells, but, avoiding excessive consumption is recommended to prevent mercury poisoning, which may cause cognitive decline.

Vitamin B3 is a crucial substance that seems to lower the risk of dementia. This vitamin is found in liver, turkey, salmon, tuna, and chicken breast. Some studies proved that vitamin B3 is involved in several vital processes inside human cells including the brain. It is also crucial for repairing damaged cell content, improve nerve qualities, lower cholesterol, and enhance blood circulation. These benefits can guard brain cells against early ageing and may delay symptoms of dementia.

Vitamin B complex is also essential for nervous integrity. They have guarding effects on nerves and blood vessels against multiple toxins. Therefore, a good intake of vitamin b complex may also be protective against dementia. This group of vitamins is found in liver, orange juice, beans, cereals, rice, eggs, and milk products.

Some theories also say that there may be a relationship between vitamin D and dementia. The role of vitamin D in decreasing the risk of dementia is still under study. Anyhow, it is advised to take enough of calcium and vitamin D to have a healthy brain.

Prevent Head injuries

Brain trauma is one common cause of increasing the risk of Alzheimer's dementia. This reason may be popular in people who enrol in frequent physical activities such as athletes as they are more prone to traumatic accidents while playing. Brain injuries during road traffic accidents are another popular cause. One advice from Alzheimer's association to prevent brain decline is to avoid head injuries by following different precautions such as wearing a seat belt while driving and wearing a helmet while playing sports including riding bikes.

Medications

Since dementia can be a result of many other health problems, good treatment of such problems using proper medications can be a great preventive measure to decrease the risks of cognitive decline. As said before, high blood pressure, diabetes type 2, and high cholesterol are all chronic disease that can harm brain cognition. Once these diseases are uncontrollable with a healthy lifestyle and dietary modification, some drugs can be used to treat them and prevent long-term probability to develop dementia. Here are few such medications used in the treatment and prevention of dementia;

- **High blood pressure Drugs**

   Uncontrolled high blood pressure has damaging effects on blood vessels. It is also a great risk factor for vascular dementia due to its involvement in developing strokes. Using drugs that lower blood pressure may be protective against dementia.

However, one study showed that having increased blood pressure later in life after the age of 80 years is less likely to be associated with dementia compared to people who never had high blood pressure.

Regardless of both suggestions, it is advised to start an active treatment plan for people who develop high blood pressure in mid-life and later after the age of 65 to minimize the danger of suffering from dementia.

- **Anti-diabetic drugs**

Type 2 diabetes, which commonly hits at mid-age (35-65) is another serious factor for vascular dementia. Therefore, a controlled level of blood sugar is needed to prevent cell injuries and other complications that might contribute to tp dementia. Once, blood glucose can't be stabilized with diet and exercises, the patients should start taking oral anti-diabetic medications which increase insulin efficacy and help controlling diabetes.

An insulin sensitizer agent called "rosiglitazone" have been found to offer additional effect in enhancing cognitive functions in patients with early Alzheimer's disease. A study on this drug found that its efficacy may be due to its role in decreasing insulin resistance, which is a major mechanism in developing diabetes. As a result, less insulin will be released to maintain the normal level of blood glucose. Insulin itself can stimulate the production of some proteins that may contribute to the progression of Alzheimer's disease as they are deposited in brain cells. Therefore, this drug may also be helpful in lowering the production of these unwanted proteins.

- **Lithium**

Lithium is a drug that may be indicated in some psychiatric disorders. Some studies discovered that lithium may be involved in minimizing the risk of Alzheimer's dementia. The mechanism of this drug in improving brain functions is by lowering the deposition of plaques of unwanted proteins that contribute to the progression of dementia and cognitive decline.

- **Steroid hormones**

It was seen that estrogen hormone may have a preventive effect on developing dementia. However, this influence can't be achieved in patients who are suffering already from cognitive decline. Estrogen enhances blood circulation to the brain and it has an anti-inflammatory role as well. This can be beneficial for improving the quality of nerve signals in the brain, which in turn can lower the risk of dementia. Furthermore, female sex hormones were found to stimulate brain regions that suffer from dementia. Intake of estrogen as a part of hormone replacement therapy can be indicated in menopause to improve symptoms and signs related to hormonal deficiency. In the same time, this can be effective in reducing the susceptibility to develop senile dementia.

- **Non-steroidal anti-inflammatory drugs (NSAIDs):**

Some studies showed that NSAIDs may be beneficial in preventing Alzheimer's dementia. Since inflammatory changes on brain play a great role in the progression of dementia, intake of NSAIDs for 2-10 years in the recommended dose seem to lower the risk of having dementia. Some inflammatory mediators are also included in the process of developing Alzheimer's dementia. Using NSAIDs stops the release of these substances protecting brain cells from further deterioration.

Aspirin is one example of NSAIDs which should be used in the average adult dose in order to achieve the desirable effects. Baby aspirin that contains lower concentration is ineffective at reducing brain decline.

Aspirin also has an additional guarding role against heart disease and high blood pressure which is another way it may help in reducing the risk of vascular dementia.

- **Vaccine:**

Production of vaccines against Alzheimer's disease is under research. Many studies depended on the idea of using the body's natural immunity to fight against the deposition of protein plaques in brain cells. this deposition may be the main reason for suffering from brain shrinkage and cognitive decline. The desired efficacy of this theory isn't accomplished yet, and no approved vaccine was found. Clinical trials found that this immunological reaction in brain cells may increase inflammatory process while lowering the deposition of unwanted plaques. However, based on the same concept, some modifications were performed as an attempt to reduce inflammation that may result from the immunological reactions. As a result, a review in the Journal of Alzheimer's disease introduced an oral vaccine to treat dementia by lowering inflammatory activities of the brain. This area is still under discussion, but the hope of receiving a treatment soon is still alive.

CHAPTER 6

Dietary Habits That Prevent Dementia

Healthy food is essential for the proper functioning of the brain cells and may play a great role in preventing several brain disorders including dementia. Many types of researches were done looking for a particular diet that may reduce the risk of dementia. No particular nutritional substance was declared to be preventive against brain decline. The reason why this wasn't accomplished is that many other influences other than food are affecting the progression of dementia and studying the role of a specific supplement may be very difficult. However, it is confirmed that a balanced diet can prevent heart diseases and diabetes which will then reassure a healthy brain.

Malnutrition in older ages is also a common problem which causes several health drawbacks and may increase the progression of dementia. Patients of dementia usually suffer from improper feeding may be due to depression, loss of appetite or due to binge drinking. As a result, they may suffer from weight loss and nutritional deficiencies accelerating cognitive decline.

Mid-life obesity is an additional risk for dementia in older ages. Dietary modification is crucial within this period of life to prevent obesity and to improve brain health and prevent dementia.

Some nutritional supplements may reduce the risk of brain deterioration. Vitamin B complex, E, D, and omega-3 are all substances that improve general health and may delay symptoms of dementia. Moreover, evidence showed that a Mediterranean diet may minimize the risk of brain deterioration and dementia.

Mediterranean diet

It is a type of diet originally started in Greece, Italy, and Spain in the previous century. It depends mainly on a high intake of fresh fruits, green vegetables, cereals and olive oil. In addition, moderate consumption of Mediterranean fish, milk products, and red wine are also included in this diet plan with decreased feeding on meats.

Depending on these principles, olive oil is the source of fat that constitutes around 25% of the total calories consumed. An essential feature of this type of diet is having a low concentration of saturated fat which forms about 8 % of the total calories. The Mediterranean diet further contains high contents of unsaturated fats and fibers. These concentrations are beneficial to brain functions. Olive oil itself contains unsaturated fats that have several health benefits.

In 2016, a study was published on the effect of Mediterranean diet on improving cognitive brain abilities. The result of this review found that there is an association between better brain performance and a Mediterranean diet.

Another study also showed that following a Mediterranean diet plan is related to a reduced risk of dementia. Adherence to this kind of diet may contribute to delaying the symptoms of Alzheimer's disease in old ages. Above all, multiple types of research found a close association between the Mediterranean diet and lowering heart disease, type 2 diabetes and cancer.

The major biological mechanisms through which this diet is associated with lower risk of brain decline include; protection against vascular events, relief of inflammation, and minimizing the oxidative stress. The protective impact on vascular system contributes to lowering the incidence of heart disease and strokes which can prevent vascular dementia. Moreover, the Mediterranean diet slows the progression of inflammatory processes by limiting several inflammatory mediators and substances involved. This action is beneficial to protect brain cells from inflammatory damage and cognitive deterioration.

Oxidative stress can be another risk for brain cell injuries and disruption of cognitive power. Mediterranean diet help relieving this stress as it is rich in vegetables, fruits, and other healthy elements that contain a high concentration of antioxidants. These antioxidants are effective in improving cellular metabolism and detoxifying toxic substances. Mediterranean diet is also found to increase the concentration of neutrophins, which are protective proteins for nerve cells against oxidative stress.

Based on several studies that discuss the relationship between the Mediterranean diet and the prevention of dementia, there are multiple evidence, that adherence to this type of food may lower the risk of Alzheimer's disease. However, treatment of a patient suffering from dementia through this diet plan wasn't found to be beneficial in improving symptoms of brain decline.

It is advised to adhere to a Mediterranean diet since mid-life to protect brain cells against deterioration and lower the incidence of cognitive decline after the age of 65.

<u>Omega-3</u>

They are polyunsaturated fatty acids (PUFA) containing alpha-linolenic acid (ALA), docosahexaenoic acid (DHA), and eicosapentanoic acid (EPA). All of these fatty acids are not synthesized inside the body, which means that they should be taken from outside sources such as oily fish. DHA is the omega-3 PUFA that constitutes brain tissues. These brain tissues are formed mainly from lipids and phospholipids. Thus, the concentration of fatty acids inside brain tissue is affected by dietary intake. Omega-3 PUFA is also essential in promoting nerve cell growth and enhancing the transmission of nerve impulses between nerve cells which is essential for an intact nervous system.

Oily fish like salmon, sardines, fresh tuna, and swordfish are the richest source of omega-3 PUFA. Moreover, other sources of these fatty acids are also available such as eggs and meats particularly if animals consume a good amount of omega-3.

The role of omega-3 in lowering the risk of dementia seems to be mediated also by the protective role they play on vascular system by reducing cholesterol levels and preventing vascular events.

Omega-3 fats are anti-inflammatory agents that decrease the severity of inflammation processes inside brain cells. Further, they are involved in reducing the deposition of unwanted proteins in brain tissues in neurodegenerative diseases. All of these effects are crucial to guard against Alzheimer's disease and vascular dementia. Regarding their effects as anti-inflammatory agents, omega-3 PUFA directly inhibits release of "cytokines" which are the messengers that trigger steps of inflammatory processes inside brain cells. As a result, brain inflammation will be reduced, lowering the risk of brain damage.

Since omega-3 fats are primary constituents of phospholipids that form membranes of nerve cells, their abundance is required for health and intact nervous system.

Omega-3 PUFA is protective against heart diseases and enhances brain circulation. They help to maintain the proper functioning of the heart which lowers the risk of developing strokes that may cause damage to brain cells. These fatty acids also improve the structure of blood vessels, which in turn is reflected in the quality of blood supply to brain tissue. Above all, they may contribute to reducing levels of blood pressure and keeping a balanced lipid and cholesterol profile which are all important to reduce the possibility of developing dementia.

Several studies and systematic reviews studied the protective role of omega-3 against cognitive decline and dementia. One published study showed that patients of dementia usually eat fewer fish and meats than others who have good cognitive functions. Consumption of oily fish in mid-life as well may be associated with better brain abilities and cognitive power. Additional evidence also states that the level of omega-3 PUFA is markedly lower in people who are suffering from dementia in contrast to other normal population in the same age. However, other factors may be associated with the guarding effects of omega-3 on brain cells. These factors include other healthy habits, educational abilities, and lifestyle.

Based on several pieces of researches, a good consumption of omega-3 is generally beneficial to brain power and cognitive abilities. Although their protective role against dementia is found, the net result depends upon other multiple factors that collaborate together towards lowering the incidence of dementia. It is recommended to regularly eat fish that are rich in omega-3 for better brain functions since childhood. This can play a protective role in developing brain deterioration while getting old and may decrease the incidence of Alzheimer's dementia after the age of 65.

<u>B vitamins</u>

Vitamin B complexes are a group of vitamins that are essential for the integrity of the nervous system and brain functions. They also play a significant role in cell metabolisms. There is a close relationship between several neurological problems and deficiency in B vitamins. These vitamins are chemical agents that can't be produced adequately inside that human body. So, they should be taken through external dietary sources.

Evidence from several studies reported that all types of Vitamin b may be involved in preventing dementia.

Vitamin B9 (also called folate) and vitamin B12 are mainly involved in protein and DNA metabolism inside cells. An inadequate concentration of these vitamins inside cells including brain cells will disrupt normal protein metabolism leading to accumulation of protein plaques which are a major mechanism in regular cognitive decline and neurodegenration in older ages. A study held in the UK found that the concentration of folate and vitamin B12 is reduced steadily while ageing. This deficiency was found to be about 5 % after the age of 65. Then it becomes 10% in people older than 75. Thus, these age group may be more prone to impaired cell metabolism and subsequently lower cognitive abilities. A good intake of these vitamins since mid-life may be protective against brain decline.

Folate can be found in broccoli, brown rice, liver, asparagus, chickpeas, and brussels sprouts, while Vitamin B12 present in a good concentration in cheese, salmon, eggs, meat, and milk.

Vitamin B6 (also called pyridoxine) plays a key role in the production of haemoglobin and substances that are responsible for the transmission of nerve signals between nerve cells. it also contributes to the metabolism of lipids and proteins inside cells.

Sources of this vitamin include; milk, eggs, potatoes, vegetables, soya beans, and fishes.

Getting an adequate supply of vitamin B complex can be a good preventive factor against dementia combined with other dietary sources that promote brain functions. It is advised to consume a sufficient amount of these substances since childhood with increased intake in the mid-life period.

Anti-oxidants

As mentioned before, oxidative stress over brain cells and neurons is a key reason for developing dementia, especially in Alzheimer's diseases. This stress can cause cell injuries that may progress to cell death. With the time, multiple damaged cells will impair functions of the brain and cognitive decline will manifest. The progression of this process increases gradually as people age because more oxidative stress will be imposed on brain cells with a lower capacity to fight against this stress. Anti-oxidants are substances that guard neurons and brain cells against damage by detoxifying the toxic substances that mediate these injuries. Some antioxidants are also specified in guarding nerve cells against damage. This means that the antioxidant diet may have a greater impact in fighting oxidative stress in the ageing brain.

These antioxidants include in multiple supplements in the form of Vitamin E, Vitamin C, and flavonoids.

Vitamin E has significant anti-oxidant function and it contributes to protecting gene translation and multiple enzymatic reactions particularly in nerve cells. it is also important for a strong immunity to fight against infections. Moreover, Vitamin E participates in the production of red blood cells and regulates the actions of vitamin K which is responsible for good blood flow and prevention of blood clotting. Some pieces of research still study the role of vitamin E against heart diseases, strokes, and dementia. This vitamin is found in olive oil, nuts, and seeds.

A study was published to describe the role of consuming food rich in antioxidants in preventing the long-term danger of dementia. Participants of this study were people aged more than 55 years that weren't suffering from symptoms of dementia and they were observed for a period of more than 9 years.

The results of this observation found that high intake of vitamin E may have a moderate effect on reducing risk of Alzheimer's disease and dementia.

Vitamin C is essential for cell growth and repair of injuries in the brain cells. It is also involved in multiple enzymatic activities inside cells and plays a role in wound healing in addition to its antioxidant activities. Similar to Vitamin E, the antioxidant role of vitamin C is crucial for maintaining a good function of body tissues including the brain. Sources of this vitamin are Broccoli, Brussel sprouts, potatoes, peppers, and orange.

Flavonoids also collaborate with vitamin c and have an anti-inflammatory role in addition to their protective function against infections. These substances can be founded in dark chocolate, grapes, citrus, berries, grains, vegetables, onions, and wine.

<u>Caffeine & coffee</u>

Several studies talked about the possible role of caffeine in brain stimulation and lowering the risk of dementia. One published study found that the blood level of caffeine in patients who developed dementia was lower than those who had normal cognitive abilities. This may be an indication that caffeine may be protective for brain cells. Furthermore, caffeinated products are known by their immediate stimulating influence on the nervous system. This effect is achieved by improving nerve signaling which increases alertness and activity of the central nervous system.

Multiple researches also discussed the probable effect of caffeine in reducing the danger to suffer from cognitive decline after the age of 65. These studies illustrated data from several participants who took regular doses of caffeine on a daily basis for a long time. The results found that coffee has the ability to decrease the risk of developing Alzheimer's disease and dementia.

Although coffee was found to improve the cognitive power of the brain, the exact mechanism of doing that is still unclear. One study talked about a component in coffee called "eicosanoyl-5-hydroxytryptamide" which may be responsible for this preventive effect against dementia. This compound was found to have neuroprotective benefits which seem to significantly lower the incidence of dementia in coffee drinkers.

The best result of using coffee as a preventive factor against cognitive decline can be achieved by regular intake of sufficient dose of coffee early in the mid-life before any cognitive decline becomes apparent. This was depicted in one study where around 1400 participants with ages from 65 to 79 drank coffee regularly and followed up for 21 years. The results showed that the risk of developing dementia decreased by around 65% in people who took 3-5 daily cups of coffee since their midlife.

More evidence showed that caffeine may also increase learning abilities and memory performances. This may be due to its effect on the hippocampus which is a structure in the brain responsible for memory and learning. Moreover, caffeine was also found to be beneficial as a treatment for dementia after developing the symptoms of brain decline. The reason for this is that caffeine has a potential role in lowering the level of inflammatory mediators reducing the intensity of inflammation.

Caffeinated Coffee raises the level of a substance called granulocyte-colony stimulating factor (GCSF) in the blood. This agent promotes the cognitive performance of the brain and stimulates the production of new connections between nerve cells.

Other ingredients inside coffee may have an additional protective role against dementia. For example, a substance called "trigonelline" was seen to have guarding effects against neurodegeneration and may enhance memory functions as well. Aeveral antioxidants are also found in coffee with a potent impact of defending the brain against cognitive decline. They play an anti-inflammatory role as well and help in maintaining a good concentration of acetylcholine, a key nerve transmitter, in the brain.

Therefore, it seems that coffee contains some beneficial components including caffeine that may lower the risk of developing dementia and protect brain cells against cognitive decline.

Superfood

It is a term that describes a group of food associated with numerous health benefits including preventive role against dementia. Superfoods include food that contains a high density of vitamins, minerals and other crucial elements for health. Berries, kiwifruit, beans, nuts, seeds, and whole grains are all examples of superfoods that provide enormous benefits to human health.

In addition, almost all superfoods contain a good concentration of antioxidants and anti-inflammatory agents which actively play a role in protecting brain cells and in preventing neurodegenerative processes in Alzheimer's disease. The fiber content of these foods is usually high and can help in assuring a healthy digestive system, balanced cholesterol profile, and low risk of serious metabolic diseases such as diabetes.

The way superfoods may protect the brain against cognitive decline can be achieved by several ways. Firstly, regular intake of superfoods provides the body with a healthy balanced diet rich in vitamins and minerals with less load of calories. As a result, there will be a lower risk of obesity and elevated cholesterol profile which in turn decrease the liability to diabetes type 2. Since obesity, increased cholesterol profile, and diabetes are all risks for developing dementia, superfoods are considered as a key factor that may reduce the risk of dementia.

The anti-inflammatory properties of superfoods are also protective against heart diseases, vascular insult, and stroke. Thus, the brain will be less vulnerable to encounter vascular disorders which may harm the brain cells.

Avocado is rich in a compound called lutein which has a specific enhancing effect on the brain. Lutein can be also found in leafy green vegetables and it is believed that eating an abundance of this substance can help in maintaining a good cognitive health of the brain.

Blueberries are common fruits in the list of superfoods. It is also considered a super fruit with several health values. Researches show that berries are protective against heart disease, different types of cancers, and can also fight against dementia. Berries contain essential substances called flavonoids that were seen to reduce the oxidative damage of the brain.

Nuts are also included in superfoods as they also contribute to enhancing the memory and reducing the risk of cognitive decline. Additional studies were also published on effects of nuts reporting that they may be able to enhance memory in patients who are already suffering from Alzheimer's dementia.

Beans are also rich in fibers which are important to reduce cholesterol profile to reduce the risk of heart diseases and diabetes.

Pomegranates are well-known fruits with multiple benefits for brain function. Recent studies also found that they have remarkable positive results in the brains of mice that suffer from Alzheimer's disease. Furthermore, regular intake of these fruits is seen to have a neuroprotective impact in mice. The same could apply to human brain.

Superfoods also include beneficial oily fishes such as salmon and sardine. As mentioned before, these fatty fishes are rich in omega-3 fatty acids which are extremely beneficial for brain cells and improve cognitive power. They also have a protective impact against heart diseases and strokes.

CHAPTER 7

Role Of Ketones In The Prevention Of Dementia

Our brain requires a greater supply of energy to perform its basic functions. This is about 20-23% of the total body's energy requirements. Glucose is the source of energy required by the brain. The recent evidence from research shows that glucose metabolism is severely affected in people with neurodegenerative diseases as if Alzheimer's disease. There is a specific pattern of glucose impairment shown in different parts of the brain. Due to this, glucose cannot adequately supply the brain with energy, instead, ketones are used. This glucose impairment is shown as a result of insulin resistance, APOE4 carriers and also in the individuals with the family history of neurodegenerative diseases as if Alzheimer's disease. This phase of impairment is named as "latent presymptomatic glucose decreased metabolism in the brain". One of the effective and easiest solutions is supplying the body with ketones so that the brain can use it for their energy metabolism. Hence, the chance of developing dementia or any other neurodegenerative and neuropsychiatric disorders are really low.

In addition, ketones are helpful in preventing the deposition of amyloid plaques, a special type of proteins deposition in the brain. The development of neurodegenerative diseases as if dementia or Alzheimer's disease as a result of the inflammatory mediators that attack our neurons and brain will thereby decrease. However, ketones have a special role in reducing these mediators. Ketones that are used up by the brain as fuel also have a neurotrophic or nerve growth effect that may cause a negative effect on the development of dementia or Alzheimer's disease.

Why does our brain prefer ketones?

When there is a problem in the glucose metabolism, our body shifts to a special state where our brain can use ketones as a form of energy. This is due to the fact that ketone bodies do not need the help of insulin to enter any cell. Also, these ketones enter the cells, especially of brain cells through an easier transport system than that of glucose transport.

Sources of ketones

Ketogenic diet

A ketogenic diet is a specialised form of diet in which carbohydrates are reduced to a low amount, while the fat consumption is increased and the protein consumption is kept at a moderate level. This low-carbohydrate state and not so high protein in the body decreases the level of insulin in the blood. It signals the fat reserves to be broken down by the body in search of energy. Hence, this special type of starvation of glucose activates the ketone metabolism especially true for the brain. The ketones are produced when there is no glucose in the body by the breakdown of glycogen in the liver. In order for the fats to be metabolised to ketones, the level of insulin should be kept at a low level. This helps to keep up the normal function of the body even during non-ketogenic diet starvation. However, as we have seen from many studies, glucose uptake by the brain decreases with age. This results in very few energy molecules reaching the brain cells. On the other hand, the ketogenic diet creates a special way in which ketones are loaded into the brain to be used as an efficient fuel. More specifically, an increase in the level of ketones in the plasma attracts the brain and the brain effectively absorbs them. Also, ketones reduce the effect of Alzheimer induced dementia. This alternate fuel store can be made just by changing the diet to a ketogenic diet.

A study conducted on 23 elderly individuals with cognitive impairment of mild degree who were started on a low carbohydrate diet for a period of 6 weeks showed greater improvement in the cognitive functions than their counterparts who were given high carbohydrate diet.

However, depriving the body of certain nutrients can have a negative effect on the overall health of the person.

Ketone supplements:

The best alternative to this is using supplements of ketones as if beta-hydroxybutyrate or use of other fats. Coconut oil can be the best source of fat that can be used. Caprilic acid is a specialised fatty acid presents in the coconut oil and they make up to 8% of the fats. These fats are readily metabolized into ketones after its absorption to the body.

High-fiber diet:

Apart from these supplements and coconut oil, fiber can be used as an alternative source of ketones generation. A high-fiber diet is another rich source of ketones. Digestible fiber is converted into fatty acids in the gut by the activity of microbes. These fatty acids are readily converted into ketones. These alternative supplements and high-fiber diet, unlike the ketogenic diet, do not have any negative effect. These supplements and the high-fiber diet also have a positive influence on the vascular and on the heart health of a person. Hence, these supplements and high-fiber diet not only fuel the brain with ketones but also eliminate the potential risk factors for the development of dementia.

Supplementation with triglyceride:

A simple way to supply our brain with ketones can be with the help of triglyceride supplements. They can replace the need for a low-carbohydrate diet or ketogenic diet. BENEFIC study tested people by giving triglyceride supplement twice a day. This supplement is a medium chain triglyceride, which contains 30g of fat per day (a Ketogenic form of fat). This study incorporated 50 individuals and they were randomly given supplement or placebo. All these individuals who were recruited to this study had mild memory decline. The possible treatment was given for a period of 6 months. After 6 months, special scans were performed on these individuals and it showed that 4-8% energy decline was associated with glucose in patients with memory impairment of mild degree.

Further, this study showed that the metabolic rate of the brain increased in individuals who were given triglyceride supplement. The effect was equal to the amount of increment of ketones in the circulation. Also, improvement in memory is noticed in people who received this supplement. This was also equal to the level of plasma ketones. This showed that 30g of triglyceride supplement matched with the two-thirds of the energy requirements of the brain showing that people do not need to restrict what they eat. Instead, they can use this supplement in their day-to-day life.

This makes the dementia prevention more easy and affordable.

A study involving 20 people with Alzheimer's disease or mild degree of cognitive impairment with triglyceride (medium chain) drink showed improvement in memory in people who are not APOE4 carriers.

Physical exercises:

Physical exercises also have a special role to play in the ketone metabolism of the brain. One study shows that physical exercise increases the uptake of the ketones by our brain. This result in the reduction of the energy deficit of the brain and hence, this property of physical exercise helps in the prevention of dementia by keeping the brain cells in a healthy state with adequate energy to perform their function.

Coconut oil:

Coconut oil is one of the important oil that is included in many researches related to dementia prevention. Coconut oil contains different types of fatty acids. Among them lauric acid, palmitic acid, caprylic acid and myristic acid are considered the most. All these acids are medium chain triglycerides. These fatty acids are one of the important sources of ketones. Hence, coconut oil is advised to be used in the prevention of diabetes of the brain or Alzheimer's disease.

One study showed that using coconut oil or Axona of 10-20g per day in the randomised trial with 152 individuals for a period of 90 days with a mild-moderate degree of Alzheimer's disease had positive effects. People who are not carriers of APOE4 had a greater positive effect on the cognitive function.

CHAPTER 8

Role Of Physical Exercises In The Prevention Of Dementia

Physical exercise plays a vital role in maintaining a healthy lifestyle. In other words, the contribution of the physical exercises to the general fitness, brain health, mental fitness, and wellness is inevitable. The benefits of physical exercises are more than bodybuilding or keeping the body in a desirable shape. Physical activities are highly important to maintain sufficient blood flow to the brain. In addition, this sufficient flow of blood provides enough oxygen and other vital nutrients to the brain cells. Hence, physical exercises indirectly help the growth and survival of the brain cells. Physical exercise takes part in cognitive improvement. This role has attracted many researchers to know the extent of physical exercise in the prevention of dementia.

Multiple researches are still conducted to know the exact relationship between physical exercise and dementia. However, many studies have shown that physical exercise performed during their entire life has a favourable effect on the prevention of dementia and also decreases the change in cognitive impairment. Apart from preventing dementia, physical exercises have a specific role in risk factor reduction. The indirect route by which dementia is prevented by the physical exercises is crystal clear. Regular physical exercises have a positive effect on heart health. Thus, stroke and other potentially dangerous heart diseases can be avoided with the help of regular exercises. Addition of physical activity also has a positive effect on the prevention and control of hypertension and diabetes mellitus of type

2. Also, physical exercises reduce the risk of obesity and further help to keep the body weight under a healthy limit. All these factors that are discussed above have a potential role in the development of cognitive impairment and pave the way to dementia. However, the chances of developing dementia with physical exercise decrease as these risk factors are modified by regular physical training. Many studies show that regular physical activity prevents dementia in the older population. While other studies show that physical exercise that performed during early, mid and late life slows the development of cognitive impairment and other changes that occur as a result of ageing.

Major benefits of physical exercises:

Exercises strengthen the cardiovascular system: A strong heart and lungs lower the blood pressure. The result is less tension in the blood vessels of the body and brain. When the motor activity of the body consumes more nitric oxide, that is, the gas that dilates blood vessels, improved blood flow is obtained. In addition, the blood flow, which increases during moderate intensity exercises, does not allow the arteries of the brain to harden.

People have had a stroke and have a history of Alzheimer's disease, demonstrate improved performance in their thinking tests when regular moderate physical exertion is carried out. Best of all, of course, start training in youth, but it's never too late to do it.

Exercises regulate the energy supply of cells: As we age, our insulin levels decrease, and it is more difficult for glucose to enter the cells to feed them with energy. Then the sugar level rises sharply, and by-products are created in the cells - for example, free radicals damage the walls of blood vessels. The result is a risk of stroke or Alzheimer's disease. But, exercise increases the blood supply to the brain and thus, brain cells get adequate nutrients to grow and survive. Thereby, exercises increase the life expectancy of our brain cells.

Exercises help fight obesity: In addition to the fact that the fat deposited in the body causes serious damage to the cardiovascular system and metabolic processes, it also has an extremely negative effect on the brain. Being overweight doubles the likelihood of developing dementia, and if accompanied with high blood pressure and cholesterol, the risk of developing senile dementia increases by 6 times.

When people retire, they begin to think that they deserve a rest after their life's work, and pay full attention to food. This results in obesity. However, physical exercises kick-start the person metabolism from sedentary to fully functional metabolism and thus, burn calories. In this way, exercises fight off obesity and keep our brain healthy. That is why it is necessary to be physically active even after your retirement from work.

Exercises increase the threshold of resistance to stress: Exercises mitigate the destructive effects of excessive cortisol levels, a chronic stress hormone, which also provokes the development of depression and dementia.

Exercises improve mood: Many scientific studies have shown that improvement in mood reduces the risk of dementia. Physical exercises allow us to stay out of our day-to-day life's problems and to stay in contact with people and make friends. Social connections are very important for a good mood. In addition, when performing exercises outdoor, nature also plays a vast role in improving the mood positively. Social engagements help humans to build new relationships, learn new information and exchange ideas and thoughts which could further improve cognitive functions of the brain.

Exercises strengthen the immune system: Stress and age decrease the immune response to external stimuli, but physical exercises strengthen it. Even moderate intensive exercises increase the antibodies and lymphocytes, which are known as T-cells in response to diseases. Antibodies fight bacterial and viral infections, and the greater presence of T-cells in the body allows it to more actively prevent cancer and resist the development of dementia.

Further, a survey conducted on the population confirms that the most stable risk of cancer is associated with constant hypodynamia or lack of movements. Physically active people, for example, have a 50% lower risk of colon cancer than who are not physically active.

Exercises strengthen the skeletal system:

Osteoporosis is not directly related to the brain, but it should always be remembered that strong bones are another necessity in the older population. As a result of physical exercise, bone strength increases and thus, the development of osteoporosis is prevented. This secures the elderly population to perform physical exercises without any difficulty.

Exercise increases motivation: As we age, the motivation within us decreases as a result of a number of changes that happens in our body during the process of ageing. When a person moves, he/she naturally increase their motivation by strengthening the connections between dopamine neurons. At the same time it protects them from another neurodegenerative disease known as Parkinson's disease. Neurodegenerative diseases increase the chance of development of cognitive impairment and dementia and with the help of exercises it is possible to prevent these conditions.

Exercise develops the neuroplasticity of our brain: The best way to protect against neurodegenerative diseases is to create a strong and healthy brain. Aerobic exercises help in strengthening the connections between nerve cells, creating more synapses for expanding the neural network and encouraging stem cells to divide more actively, turning into full-fledged functional neurons. The stronger the neural connections, the better the brain will prepare for any negative effects that it may encounter. This is very much essential in the ageing population. Improved neuroplasticity stimulated by physical exercises strengthen the brain and keep human brain away from cognitive impairment and dementia.

Regular exercising

Regular exercising should be well understood in order to understand the standard practice and also to benefit from dementia. There are no specific parameters that define regular physical activeness, but a regular exercise should be performed for long-term and with a frequent consistency. For example, 20-30 minutes of aerobic exercises per session. Any exercise that can increase the heart rate and supply sufficient oxygen to the brain is called as an effective exercise that can influence the body positively. More theoretically, the oxygen consumption per unit time values is an indicator of the beneficial property of physical exercise on the body's fitness level. The higher the value of oxygen consumption per unit time, the greater the effectiveness of the exercise will be and favours better fitness and wellbeing. The consistency, long-term exercise and the oxygen consumption per unit time value can nearly define how regular you should exercise. The regular exercise of the above-mentioned nature has beneficial properties in preventing dementia and also reducing the risk factors. Non-consistent or less frequent exercises have no evidence in the prevention of dementia.

How do we choose the right exercise?

Generally, three types of regular exercises are indicated in order to achieve general fitness. The types of exercises are,

Aerobic exercises - These are a specialized form of exercises that are performed for a longer duration at a moderate intensity. The main aim of this exercise is to improve the general fitness as well as brain health by increasing the blood supply to the brain. The duration and the intensity of these exercises can be increased slowly. However, 30 min of aerobic exercises at least 3-4 times a week is minimally indicated to produce a beneficial outcome. The most common types of aerobic form of exercises are swimming, jogging, walking, dancing and cycling. These exercises are easier to perform and have minimal chance of injury.

Strength training - Work with weights or resistance devices twice a week. Each time perform at least three sets with the repetition of 10-15 times each set. This exercise helps to prevent osteoporosis. These exercises are scientifically proven to reduce the chances of osteoporosis and also increases bone strength. Having strong bones will ensure that you are able to perform other exercises to maintain the good health of the brain. It is always better to have a personal trainer when doing strength training or weight training exercises. This helps to avoid unnecessary injuries.

Balance and flexibility exercises - It is very much important to perform these exercises twice a week for at least 30 minutes. Yoga, Pilates, Tai Chi (Tai Chi), martial arts and dance are the most common balance and flexibility exercises. These develop skills to maintain balance and flexibility, which is important for mobility and quickness. The skills that are achieved from balance and flexibility exercises help to achieve more efficient results with aerobic and strength training exercises. For self-training, use a large rubber ball or various kinds of balancing boards (discs) or the Bosu ball with a flat base: it is convenient to hold the balance on it while straining the abdominal muscles and buttocks.

It is important to seek advice from a doctor on what type and intensity of exercises are best suited. This varies from individual to individual. Usually, planned and supervised exercise programs are ideal, but any exercise is beneficial to the body. If appropriate facilities are not available, it is always possible to adapt to what is available, and of course to benefit from simpler kinds of exercise such as walking. Other activities, such as dancing, can be a part of an exercise program. It is important that the exercise chosen has to be enjoyable and can be incorporated into day-to-day life. This makes people to perform exercises every day and to maintain physical and brain fitness at a very higher level.

Tips for safer exercise routine:

- Always warm up before beginning your exercise routine, and cool down at the end of the exercise routine.

- Start with shorter sessions and increase the repetition gradually.

- Try water activities, such as water aerobics. These are often easier on the joints and require less balance. Thus, water aerobics reduces unnecessary injuries.

- Work out in a safe environment; avoid slippery floors, poor lighting, floor rugs, and other potentially dangerous objects that can cause injury or disturb the exercise.

- If there are any difficulties in maintaining balance, exercise with something to grab onto.

- If there is any pain or feeling unwell during the exercise is a sign to immediately stop that exercise and seek medical attention.

- Last, but not least. Choose exercises that are enjoyable and which gives joy. Some of the commonly used exercises by most of the people are swimming, gardening, Tai chi, walking and water aerobics.

Scientific evidence of dementia prevention by regular physical activities

Canadian scientists claim that they traced an interesting pattern during their study with people walking at least six miles (about ten kilometres). It showed that these people who regularly walked six miles had a lower age-related loss of brain mass. At the beginning of a long-term study, its authors turned to three hundred subjects with a request to record how far they travel during regular walks. Nine years after the beginning of the observation, a brain scan was made with an assessment of its volume. After another four years, participants completed tests to assess the state of cognitive functions. So it was found that people who were walking about 10–15 km per week in old age were less susceptible to brain diseases caused by an age-related decrease in its volume, in particular, dementia. The risk of developing dementia decreased markedly, by about two times.

Another confirmation of the benefits of properly organized physical activity in the fight against senile dementia was obtained by American scientists. They surveyed elderly people aged 60 to 75 years old, who walked at a fast pace for 45 minutes a day three times a week, and found that such exercises made it possible to improve not only physical but also intellectual health. Positive changes turned out to be noticeable even against the background of the results of the control group, the participants of which were engaged in stretching indoors and doing exercises to increase the overall tone. In this regard, the importance for the aerobic exercises and practices that activate cellular processes in the brain cause an increase in the volume of grey matter is particularly emphasized.

An interesting observation was made by scientists from Chicago during the observation of a group of 970 elderly patients (mean age 80 years). It turned out that in elderly people with developed muscles, the risk of developing moderate cognitive disorders and the onset of dementia is approximately 60% lower than that of their peers. According to one interpretation, cognitive disorders and weakening of muscles have a common cause - for example, damage to the mitochondria involved in the processes of energy production in cells. Both muscle and brain can suffer from a decrease in energy production. According to another version, health problems (such as stroke or nervous system disorders) lead to muscle weakness, and therefore muscle degradation can be considered as a potential symptom of developing dementia. Another assumption is based on the opinion that physical activity as part of a healthy lifestyle allows a person to maintain a healthy brain even at an older age. One way or another, many experts stress that good physical fitness is an important condition for normal brain function.

Danish scientists first proved that intense aerobic exercise helps prevent dementia in Alzheimer's patients. The results of the study were presented by Dr. med. Günchild Waldemar, Director of the Danish Research Dementia Institute (Danish Dementia Research Center) at the first congress of the European Academy of Neurology (Europe Academy of Neurology). Scientists conducted a large-scale study of 200 patients in eight clinics in Denmark, who receive drugs for the prevention of dementia for at least three months. All patients were divided into three groups according to the amount of physical activity and were observed for 2.5 years. A special psychological test showed that 66 patients in the group who regularly exercised had significant cognitive improvements. Dr. Waldemar argues that scientists do not intend to dwell on these results and plan to take samples of patients' blood plasma before and after training to study various biological markers. In his opinion, this will help to detect the physiological mechanisms underlying the positive effect of physical exertion on patients with Alzheimer and dementia.

Physical exercise helps maintain mental acuity and can even cause an increase in the size of the hippocampus, which is a part of the brain that is responsible for emotion and long-term memory. In many people, the hippocampus tends to decrease with age, which entails some weakening of mental abilities. And physical exercises, as shown by the results of one experiment, can contribute to an increase in the size of hippocampus, even if performed irregularly. Every second of the 120 participants in the experiment performed aerobic exercises from time to time, and by the end of the experiment, the size of the hippocampus in these subjects increased by an average of 2%.

Yes, one might think that 2% is not so much, but it is just by so much that the hippocampus dries out in a year or two. Even 2 % is a considerable amount when it comes to dementia prevention. In those experiment participants who did not exercise, the hippocampus decreased by 1.4%. In other words, aerobics helps not only to prevent the loss of a part of the brain but even to increases it.

Physical exercises are an incredibly powerful means of preventing dementia and other neurodegenrative diseases. These exercises are much more effective than all drugs taken together.

CHAPTER 9

Stress and Dementia

Stress causes serious damage to our body including our brain. A study conducted shows that pathological anxiety and long-term stress can lead to degenerative changes and dysfunction of prefrontal cortex and hippocampus. These are parts of the brain that are responsible for emotions, thinking and memory, especially of long-term memory. These changes lead to dementia and depression.

Further, chronic stress has a direct effect on the immune system, heart, blood vessels and even on the metabolism. All these can contribute to the damage of brain by the long-term stress.

In another study, scientists have found that severe stress increases inflammation in the hippocampus - the brain's memory centre, which accelerates the death of neurons. All of this threatens memory deterioration in the future, according to an article published in Metabolic Brain Disease. It is known that the hippocampus is involved in the processes associated with the consolidation and preservation of long-term memories. According to scientists, this area of the brain is particularly sensitive to various forms of stress. The hippocampal nerve cells are constantly regenerating, and it is less affected than other parts of the brain by "oxygen starvation" (after the circulation stops, its neurons die not immediately, but after a few dozen minutes). At the same time, the hippocampal nerve cells die much more frequently and are more susceptible to neurodegeneration than other neurons.

Scientists have suggested that this may be due to the fact that the neurons of the memory centre are more vulnerable to various inflammatory processes in the brain that develop under the influence of stress.

In another study, it was found that during the period of stress in the hippocampus of rodents accumulated stress hormones corticosteroids. Under their influence, inflammatory processes in this area of the brain developed earlier than in other parts. According to researchers, this is due to the increased sensitivity of the hippocampal neurons to stress hormone molecules.

It was striking that even when the sources of stress disappeared, the inflammation in the brain of animals did not stop. So, even a month after the end of the experiments, the level of molecules in the hippocampus associated with inflammatory processes continued to remain extremely high. According to researchers, the consequences of this may be sad. It turns out that the cessation of chronic stress in itself does not save the hippocampus from the onset of damage. And since the hippocampus suffers from stress in the first place, it threatens to further develop dementia and emotional disturbances.

Another study conducted shows that veterans who were diagnosed with post-traumatic stress disorder (PTSD) have the likelihood of developing dementia doubled. All these studies show that how dangerous is stress to the brain health. Long-term stress should be eliminated with the help of special stress prevention techniques.

Stress and dementia prevention:

Yoga and meditation are good for the brain because they improve memory and protect against dementia. According to American scientists, yoga and meditation were more effective than exercises for memory training.

The study, which lasted three months, was attended by 25 volunteers over 55 years old. So, 11 participants once a week attended a memory training session that lasted an hour. They also performed exercises for the development of memory daily for 20 minutes. Another 14 volunteers once a week for an hour did Kundalini yoga in a group and spent 20 minutes of meditation at home Kirtan Kriya every day.

In India, Kirtan Kriya meditation has long been considered one of the ways to prevent cognitive impairment in the elderly. It includes chants, hand movements, and visualization of light.

So, after 12 weeks, experts noticed that the volunteers from both groups had improved verbal memory. That is, they have become better memorize words and names. But the visual-spatial memory, which helps to navigate in space, has noticeably improved among the participants engaged in yoga and meditation.

CHAPTER 10

Role Of Hormones On The Cognitive Function

A number of hormones participate in the regulation of cognitive processes, both in normal and pathological conditions.

Thyroid hormones

Numerous studies over the past decades have convincingly proved the role of thyroid hormones in the process of differentiation of the human brain in the prenatal period, as well as their controlling function in the process of growth of dendrites and axons, development of synapses, neuron migration, myelination, which is the basis of brain differentiation in the final periods of development. A study on cognitive functions in adolescents showed a direct correlation between long-term and spatial memory with the level of thyroxin in the mother's blood during pregnancy, while the administration of thyroid hormones (thyroxine (T4) - 90%, triiodothyronine (T3) - 10%)) prevents problems of memory, speed of thinking, and concentration. These studies show the role of thyroid hormone on the cognitive function and a thyroid hormone imbalance during old age poses potential threat to the cognitive function of the elderly population. The best possible way to prevent cognitive function decline following thyroid hormone imbalance is thyroid hormone replacement or correction therapy. This strengthens the cognitive function.

<u>Pituitary hormones</u>

Recently, numerous data have been accumulated indicating that the functions of the pituitary hormones are not limited to the regulation of peripheral processes in the body, but also have an active influence on the neuropsychic mechanisms. In particular, adrenocorticotropic hormone (ACTH) fragments and vasopressin hormone accelerate learning, stimulate attention and the process of memory consolidation, which is the transition of short-term memory to long-term. At the same time, positive effect in the correction of cognitive functions was achieved in the use of the desglycinamide analogue of vasopressin and dezamino-D-arginine vasopressin, in which hormonal effects are significantly less than that of vasopressin itself.

Prolactin, actively produced during many physiological processes in both men and women, has numerous effects on almost all organs and systems. As one of the endogenous peptide hormones of the pituitary gland, the secretion of which is under the control of the dopaminergic, GABAergic, serotonergic mechanisms, prolactin has an activating effect on the biological molecules that are secreted in the brain. Prolactin activates the processes associated not only with the parental instinct, but also with successful learning, takes part in the emergence of new interneuronal connections, as well as in the mechanism of formation of long-term memory.

Sex hormones

According to a number of researchers, the female sex hormone estrogen can also have a beneficial effect on memory. Experimental data on the prevention of estrogen cell death in the hippocampus were obtained. We describe the widespread cognitive disorders in menopausal syndrome, manifested by decreased memory, mental performance and productivity, ability to plan activities, as well as the speed of switching attention. It has been established that changes in Alzheimer's disease as a down-regulation of nuclear alpha-estrogen receptors mediating hippocampus-dependent cognitive functions are accompanied by a deficiency in the level of local estrogens and a decrease in the activity of the signaling pathway of alpha estrogen receptors. The obtained results substantiate several pathogenesis mechanisms in Alzheimer's-type dementia.

Now an increasing role in the development of central symptoms in this pathology, in particular cognitive impairment, is given to the weakening of cholinergic processes. According to the latest data, the natural age-related decline in their activity is aggravated by the growing estrogen deficiency, which increases the risk of dementia in women with severe menopausal syndrome. At the same time, estrogen deficiency forces an age-related decline in the biosynthesis of vasopressin, the "memory peptide," synthesized in the hypothalamus and plays a key role in the consolidation process. It has been established that women with insufficient estrogen synthesis can suffer from memory loss, which is completely leveled with the introduction of hormone replacement therapy (HRT). Both female and male HRT can improve memory, but there is a difference in which aspects of memory are improved. According to the data obtained by researchers, in women, estrogen administration improves verbal and visual memory, as well as attention. In men, female sex hormones can only improve verbal memory.

Meanwhile, it is known that estrogen deficiency is accompanied by a decrease in the content of the high-density lipoprotein fraction (HDL), which has an anti-atherogenic effect, and simultaneously increase the content of low-density lipoprotein (LDL). At the same time, the procoagulant and antifibrinolytic activity increases: the level of fibrinogen, VII of clotting factor, inhibitor of plasminogen activator type I and other changes that increase the coagulant activity of the blood increases. In addition to the above, estrogen deficiency is one of the factors for the formation of arterial hypertension, which, in turn, together with atherogenic activation and impaired hemostasis, increase the risk of cognitive impairment in dementia.

A decrease in the male sex hormone testosterone is also accompanied by a decrease in cognitive functions (memory and attention). It was found that the introduction of testosterone in men aged 70–80 years is characterized by an improvement in short-term memory to the level of 35–40-year-old people. However, data available in the studies on the correction of cognitive functions of testosterone-containing drugs are few and need further development.

The reproductive hormones, which also affect the state of cognitive activity, are under research. These researches include dehydroepiandrosterone (DHEA) and its sulfated form - dehydroepiandrosterone sulfate (DHEA-S). Recently, it is considered that for cognitive activity an age-related decrease in DHEA-S level is much more important than a decrease in testosterone levels. Quite a lot of research has been done on animals, mainly in rats and mice, which resulted in the following biological effects of DHEA-S: memory enhancement, antidepressant effect, and withdrawal of fear, panic, reduction of aggression. It is known that the low level of DHEA disrupts the functionality of synaptic contacts of neurons, as well as their differentiation. DHEA-S replacement therapy in the elderly, carried out for a long time (up to a year or longer), uniquely improves the processes of memory and cognition. The mechanism for improving memorization under the influence of DHEA-S, as confirmed by studies, is realized through its antagonistic effect on GABA receptors of certain brain structures, as well as an increase in the cholinergic function of the hippocampus, and its neuroprotective effect of DHEA is based on the hippocampus. Clinical studies on the use of DHEA in the correction of cognitive functions have confirmed its ability to influence mnemonic functions. Thus, an electroencephalographically-established increase in the rapid movement of the eyes during sleep in healthy volunteers with a single pharmacological dose of 500 mg of DHEA, 1 hour before sleep, is characteristic of the activation of brain areas, associated with the storage of memory. This allowed researchers to justify the potential use of DHEA to inhibit the development of senile dementia. A number of studies have shown the development of dementia against the background of a decrease in the level of circulating DHEA-S. However, no direct correlation was found between the decrease in DHEA-S production and the severity of dementia.

Of particular interest is the relationship between DHEA-S and Alzheimer's disease and other forms of dementia. A number of studies have shown the development of dementia against the background of a decrease in circulating DHEA-S. However, no direct correlation was found between the decrease in DHEA-S production and the severity of dementia. Nowadays, the role of DHEA as a protector of degenerative changes in brain neurons, which are most characteristic of Alzheimer's disease, is generally recognized. Of particular interest is the relationship between DHEA-S and Alzheimer's disease and other forms of dementia. A number of studies have shown the development of dementia against the background of a decrease in circulating DHEA-S. However, no direct correlation was found between the decrease in DHEA-S production and the severity of dementia. Now, the role of DHEA as a protector of degenerative changes in brain neurons, which are most characteristic of Alzheimer's disease, is generally recognized.

Leptin

The hormone leptin, the main hormone of adipose tissue, regulates body weight and energy expenditure by activating receptors in the hypothalamus, is one of the regulators of cognitive activity. It's possible anti-apoptotic effect is realized, which is realized by neuroblasts, osteoblasts, T-lymphocytes. Leptin is also traditionally regarded not only as a mediator affecting energy metabolism and controlling hunger and the development of overweight, but also as a risk marker for hemorrhagic stroke, coronary atherosclerosis and associated acute myocardial infarction and ischemic stroke. Some cardiovascular effects of leptin are discussed: sympathetic activation, pressor effects, vascular regulation, insulin resistance, increased platelet aggregation, proangiogenic effect. The neuroprotective effects of leptin in ischemic brain damage were investigated. Thus, a decrease in the volume of cerebral infarction caused by occlusion of the middle cerebral artery, with the administration of different doses of leptin intraperitoneally, has been shown. It may be a prospect for its use for the treatment of ischemic stroke. A study of changes in leptin levels revealed an association with physical activity, smoking, and cardiovascular diseases in history. No association with alcohol consumption, blood pressure, cholesterol, glucose and white blood cells has been identified. In addition, scientists have discovered a connection between the hormone leptin and the brain area that controls memory and the learning process. It is also known that women with a long history of depression have elevated level of leptin.

CHAPTER 11

Sex and Dementia

Sex is one of the most complex and intimate actions of a human being. It is not only associated with pleasure and reproduction but has an important role to play in the physical, mental and emotional fitness of a person. Sex is one of the complete body workouts. Sex is even more powerful than a person getting into the gym. There is no shame about having sex at even in the 60s. The involvement in regular sexual activities among elderly population shows improved mental fitness. Many scientists were interested in knowing the influence of regular sex on the cognition.

Scientists have long wanted to understand how to slow the deterioration of cognitive functions during ageing. Mental, physical, and social activities are thought to have a positive effect on brain function, as well as reducing the level of inflammation and the risk of cardiovascular and cerebrovascular diseases.

Now a new factor has been discovered that has a beneficial effect on the brain by scientists from the universities of Coventry and Oxford and it is recognized as - regular and frequent sex. This British study involved 73 people, 28 of them were men and 45 of them were women between the age ranges of 50-83.

All these individuals were assessed with the help of a questionnaire. In the questionnaire, they were asked about the general state of health, lifestyle and, most importantly, about the frequency of sexual activity in the last 12 months. The answers were provided for both the absence and frequent activity - monthly or weekly. In the term of sexual activity, researchers included not only sexual intercourse but also other sexual activities, for example, masturbation. The participants underwent tests to measure various patterns of brain activity: attention, memory, thinking, speech, and visual-spatial perception (2D and 3D views).

In order to evaluate the fluency of speech and cognitive work, the participants of the study were asked to name the maximum number of animals they can recollect within the period of 60 seconds and tell as many words as possible beginning with the letter F within 60 seconds. The subjects also copied a complex graphic pattern to evaluate the visual-spatial perception ability. For a clearer assessment of the correlation of cognitive function and sexual activity, scientists made corrections for age, gender, history of cardiovascular diseases and education.

According to the questionnaire, 37 subjects had sex weekly, 26 had sex every month, and 10 had no sexual activity. Scientists noted that this latter group consisted only of women and that such a result can be attributed both to the fact that women are less willing to talk about sex and to the fact that women become widows earlier than men. Cognitive tests showed that frequent sexual activity had the most effect on the fluency.

In addition, the most sexually active people coped better with visual-spatial tasks. The tests did not reveal differences in memory and attentive functions.

Researchers believe that the secretion of dopamine and oxytocin should be paid attention to explain the results obtained in future studies, since these biological secretions may affect the relationship between sexual activity and brain function. Therefore, these biological secretions are the target of further research.

A study which was conducted as a continuation of work in 2016 showed that sexually active older people score more points in cognitive tests than sexually inactive ones.

In the new work, however, attention was focused precisely on the parameter of the frequency of sexual activity, and to evaluate it, more tests were used. The tests used are focused on evaluating the executive function as well as the memory. Men in this study showed greater results with executive functions and memory, while women who were participated showed improved memory. Executive function and memory are important domains of cognitive function of an individual.

With each new research, we are slowly approaching an understanding of why this association exists at all, what are the underlying mechanisms, and whether the relationship between sexual activity and cognitive function in older people is causal. People do not like to think that the elderly also have sex, but we need to question this concept at the social level and see what impact sex has on people 50 years and older than already known effects on sexual health and well-being in general population who are at a younger age. These studies show the need for the abolition of social awkwardness among the general population regarding the sex life of elderly population.

CHAPTER 12

New approaches to the Prevention of Dementia

Brain training/Cognitive training/Intellectual training

This is a program of mental activities done regularly with the aim of maintaining or improving the cognitive abilities of the person being trained. The idea of brain training was started off on the assumption that just as physical fitness can be improved upon by exercising the body, we can also improve our cognitive abilities or maintain it by exercising the brain.

This assumption is being made in the light of the well established fact that aspects of our brain function remains malleable throughout life and also that a high level of mental activity are linked with lessened risks of dementia in old age. The theory is strong and support for the concept with research is still growing. An important observation that has been made in research is amongst individuals who work complex jobs or individuals who regularly engage in activities such as puzzles, crosswords or learning new hobbies throughout life. Such people seem to have lower rates of dementia and cognitive dysfunction.

Observational studies suggests some positive things with regards to this (observational studies are studies done on a group of people with the aim of finding an association between two or more factor in those people). Results from several observational studies indicate that middle-aged and the elderly people who engage in cognitively stimulating activities could have lower risk of dementia. However, these types of studies are not strong enough to tell us without doubt that the brain training activities those groups of people engaged in are directly responsible for low rates of dementia observed in them. Those people could be doing other things or may have had other interventions that led to their low rates of dementia. This is why interventional studies are important. Interventional studies are also referred to as "clinical trials" which is a term that has been used severally in this book. In clinical trials an 'intervention' is made which means that something new is introduced to the subjects by the experimenter and then the subjects are observed to see the outcome. For example, a group of individuals can be asked to start doing a new cognitive training activity and they would be followed up over time to see the effect that the new activity would have on their brain function.

There aren't much interventional studies studying the effects of sudoku or crosswords on dementia risk in older people but a number of them have studied the effect of computer brain training games. Majority of these studies sampled a small number of participants and followed up the participants for a short time. In essence these studies may not be sufficient to convince us but they do show something positive about the benefits of cognitive training which can be learnt from. It may be totally necessary to wait for bogus studies before implementing a change or learning from these little studies.

A review of 51 interventional studies indicates that brain training can produce measurable improvements in thought processing and memory ability in elderly individuals. However, the analysis revealed that elderly people who were not supervised during use of the brain training tools had no measurable improvement in their thought processing and memory. Several deductions can be made from this. It could be mean that any elderly who is to undergo brain training may need a neuropsychologist because they cannot use the tools properly to their benefit if they are not supervised. It could also mean that those that were not supervised did not do the training at all.

Computer brain training was conducted on almost 7,000 people who were above the age of 50. The brain training tool used in this study tested the reasoning and problem solving skills of the subjects. The outcome was that using this brain training tool resulted in gains in reasoning and improvement in ability to recall words noticed up to six months after completion of training. Participants were more likely to see better improvements in these brain functions the more they finished the exercises.

The benefits of using the brain training tools went beyond the functions the researchers observed. Subjects above 60 years reported an improvement in their ability to get on with their daily activities. Daily activities they did regularly such as cooking meals, managing a household budget, shopping and using public transport all became easier to handle.

For a while now, individuals that suffer from disabling traumatic brain injuries relearn how to make decisions, walk and talk with the aid of neuropsychologists. The neuropsychologists use several interventions including computer assisted cognitive exercises and games. Once before, these computer exercises were not available to the public and not everyone in need of abilities retraining could afford a neuropsychologist. However things have changed a lot today as there are a variety of commercial systems that has made computer based cognitive training games readily available for anyone to utilize. So not everyone needs to see a neuropsychologist if

The individual knows what his /her need is and can identify the right tool to use. These brain training games have shown proven gains in improving visual attention, processing speed, attention and mood in people with dementia. A successful video game trial methodology which has been used to illustrate the usefulness of this therapy goes thus; an affected person plays a video game they love for 1 hour and as frequently as 5 times a week for 3 months. That produces a total game play of 60 minutes for that 3 month period. Clinically measurable gains can be found in such people 3 months after. The cognitive gains have been found to be more pronounced in those 4 areas earlier mentioned (visual attention, mood, processing speed, attention).

A video game called was shown to reduce risk of dementia amongst about 2000 subjects who were followed up for up to 10 years. The game involved bringing pictures to the view of the subject and quickly removing the picture from their field of view and asking them to identify what was in the picture. Another tasking aspect of the game was bringing 2 pictures to the subject's field of view, one object in the patients' central visual field and the other in the peripheral field such that it is difficult to identify both of them quickly. This study is referred to as double decision. This form of processing is called speed processing and could possibly show benefits in the subjects up 10 years after using the program.

The proportion of those who participated in the training and then later had dementia was significantly smaller than those who did not receive any cognitive training.

Non Steroidal Anti-inflammatory Drugs (NSAIDs)

Research suggests an important role for the usefulness of NSAIDs in preventing dementia. Aspirin and non-aspirin NSAIDs have been researched extensively and have been found to be sometimes useful for prevention of dementia. Such NSAIDs include celecoxib, diclofenac, ibuprofen, ketoprofen, ketorolac, indomethacin, piroxicam, naproxen. NSAIDs work by reducing the production of prostaglandins in the body. Prostaglandins are the family of chemical substances that enable inflammatory reactions in the body, they aid healing, produce pain, aid blood clotting, protect the stomach mucosa, produce fever in the body. Cyclooxygenase (COX); an enzyme within the body cells is what produces prostaglandins. NSAIDs work by inhibiting COX thus reducing prostaglandin production throughout the body. A significant way, by which dementia results, is through the formation of multiple little infarcts (dead tissue) in the brain. Multiple infarcts (lacunar infarcts) is typical of vascular dementia for example. The anti clotting effect and anti inflammatory effect of NSAIDs comes to play here by preventing the formation of dead brain tissue from little clots in vessels. NSAIDs are also important for treatment of Alzheimer's disease because Alzheimer's hardly occurs in isolation without vascular dementia. At least two years of use of NSAIDs is proven to be needed to produce observable effects in prevention of dementia. Physicians may not use it as NSAIDs come with their own adverse effects but the benefit of NSAIDs with regards to dementia is proven.

Peroxisome proliferator-activated receptor (PPAR) agonists

These are drugs commonly utilized in the treatment of symptoms of the metabolic syndrome,they help in lowering serum glucose and triglyceride. There are 4 agonist types namely: alpha, delta, gamma and pan agonists. The alpha and gamma agonists have been found to produce more beneficial effects in prevention of dementia. PPAR agonists can reduce chronic inflammation and hence protect neuronal cells. When these receptors are activated, they maintain the blood brain barrier in normal state of function. They also reduce the amyloid beta (Aβ) protein induced neurotoxicity. When the PPAR-gamma receptor subtype is activated, it is able to maintain the carbohydrate and lipid content of the cells hence it balances the energy status in the brain of Alzheimer's disease patients. The fibrates act on the PPAR-alpha receptors and through their action maintains good lipid levels which helps prevent atherosclerosis. Examples of the fibrates include:clofibrate, fenofibrate, gemfibrozil, ciprofibrate, bezafibrate. Activation of the PPAR-gamma receptor helps prevent diabetes. Newer areas of research are into the production of agonists that can produce anti-diabetic as well as triglyceride lowering effects. These are the pan agonists of which some drugs exist. Resveratrol and other phenols have been found to exhibit such activity on the PPAR receptor. Having a single drug with such effects including neuroprotective effects would aid patient compliance with medications as they would not have to take too many pills at once.

Beta Amyloid (Aβ) Protein Aggregation inhibitors

Amyloid beta Aβ protein aggregates is a hallmark feature of dementia and research is still been done on creating small drug molecules that can be used to eliminate this aggregation. Baicalin has been explained before as a supplement that helps in this regard which is impressive. But more needs to be done so that doctors and scientists would be less worried about accumulating plaques as those plaques can be eliminated with a drug. Inhibiting Aβ protein aggregation has proven very difficult and challenging but investigatorsare searching wide for possible solutions. Amongst these are research endeavours aimed at activating efflux pumps in the blood brain barrier, increasing the activation of Aβ protein degradation enzymes, immunomodulation and immunotherapy targeted at Aβ protein species.

Efforts are also being made in order to inhibit the production of Aβ protein from amyloid precursor protein (APP) its precursor. These strategies also include developing β-secretase modulators and the inhibitors, and a-secretase stimulators. The strategy is also aimed at targeting pathways which affect APP1metabolism.

Neuro Protective Proteins

In addition to the Aβ protein innovations, some work is also being done in the aspect of antioxidation and anti-inflammatory early in the disease. This is not just about Alzheimer's disease but also other neurodegenerative diseases as well. For instance, there is a small peptide which was derived from a neuroprotective protein which is a drug candidate that has been shown to protect neuronal cells from Aβ-induced insults. Additionally, researchers are working towards developing peptidomimetic compounds which help activate neurotrophin receptors and hence protect neurons from cellular death. Other developments that increase the receptor signalling of brain-derived neurotrophic receptor (BDNF) have shown promising results in non human primates.Some effects seen includerestoration of cognitive function and protectionof the neurons from death.

Dimebon

This is an antihistamine manufactured in Russia. The generic name is latrepirdine. It has been tried severally as a possible nootropic (substance that aids neural health) in humans but more studies are still needed to establish its beneficial effect. It has only been shown to have neuro protective effects in mice and has shown some little positive effects in preliminary tests done in humans. It has not yet passed successfully through a clinical trial which is why the drug is still being researched into. The drug is thought to function through stabilisation of the mitochondria.

Regeneration

Researchers are keenly looking into this field to help regenerate patients' cells. This will help regain lost functionality that occurred due to damage of neurons. Options for this with current research include induction of pathways that aid the stimulation of neurogenesis or introduction of exogenous stem cells.

Conjugated Oestrogen

Some studies have shown that oestrogen replacement therapy given to women who have entered menopause enables them to improve in their cognition. It was also seen that the therapy prevents development of dementia. But some studies differ on this stance and claim that oestrogen does not produce any cognitive related benefit in asymptomatic women, stating that cognition may tend to improve in post menopausal women who are given oestrogen due to the fact that their menopausal symptoms have been cured. However neurophysiologic and biochemistry studies have shown some ways through which oestrogen produces its benefit especially with regards to dementia. In some areas of the brain, oestrogen produces an increase in the cholinergic and serotonergic activity, the neural circuitry is maintained, and there is beneficial lipoprotein regulation and prevention of reduced blood supply to the brain matter. In observational studies and trials studying the effect of oestrogen on cognitive function in postmenopausal women without dementia, it is observed that cognition tends to improve in peri-menopausal women. Meta-analysis of observational studies that measured the effect of oestrogen use on the risk of dementia developing in post menopausal women showed a 29% decreased risk of developing dementia in them but the findings of the studies are heterogeneous. Due to the risks associated with oestrogen therapy, oestrogen is not routinely prescribed but it has strong benefits for post menopausal women. A good understanding of the oestrogen hormone neurobiology is still needed for high effectiveness to be achieved. It is also necessary for the hormone to be prescribed in the correct formulation, at the right time and to the correct population of women.

Active immunization and Passive immunization

Vaccines against Alzheimer's disease in particular have been formulated and have been proven to be beneficial. Active immunization is often used in the context of preventing diseases from germs. What happens in active immunization is that a very little amount of a germ or a harmless form of a germ is introduced into the body. The body's immune system reacts to the presence of that germ and attacks it. Because the germ is very little or very harmless the body deals with it easily. But in the process of getting rid of the germ the immune system is also stimulated to produce some immune cells that are specialized to attack that germ or the immune system is stimulated to produce some cells that can identify the germ very quickly the next time it comes into the body so that it can be quickly eliminated. Passive immunization on the other hand is just like creating a drug that is very specific for a germ. Antibodies that can attack a germ are cloned in an equine or in the laboratory; the antibodies are then extracted, purified then put up for sale in a pharmacy. These synthetically prepared antibodies bear semblance to the antibodies your body would produce when faced with that germ. The idea behind inventing dementia vaccines is borne out of the fact that Alzheimer's disease is accompanied by neuropathologies characterized macroscopically by diffuse brain atrophy, and microscopically by senile plaques (SPs), neurofibrillary tangles (NFTs) and neuronal loss in the brain. Vaccines have been proven to be beneficial in eliminating those microscopic pathologies by preparing the immune system in advance to meet with these problems in the case of active immunization or by injecting the patient with antibodies that can help cure the condition as is in the case of passive immunization. This is a significant milestone although a lot more still needs to be done to ensure these vaccines are safe and that these vaccines produce consistent results in humans. SPs are formed from by extracellular deposits of β amyloid, and at a later stage SPs are accompanied by inflammatory responses from other cells like the microglia and astrocytes in the brain. The amyloid B protein aggregates are derived from the amyloid precursor protein (APP). A lot of useful knowledge pertaining to the way amyloid proteins are formed led to the postulation of the amyloid cascade hypothesis which just tells us how these SPs come about and gives us ideas on how to tackle them. This has led to new preventive and therapeutic strategies targeting the amyloid cascade being established regularly. Most immunization models with Aβ protein showed improvement in cognitive functions and reduced Aβ plaque pathology. The vaccination therapy for Alzheimer's was invented by Dale Schenk et al. They started by immunizing young mice with Aβ protein with adjuvant and found that the amyloid deposits were significantly reduced when those immunized mice were examined at a later time. They also found that immunization of the mice with Aβ at an age when they had started having amyloid deposits in their brains reduced amyloid plaques and prevented more amyloid proteins from being deposited. They also saw that a similar effect was produced by injection of monoclonal/polyclonal Aβ antibodies (passive immunization).The immunized mice showed improvement. A clinical trial of active immunization done on humans used Alzheimer's patients in the United Kingdom. However, 6% of the patients developed a sub-acute meningoencephalitis (a brain inflammatory disease) after one to three injections of the vaccine into their muscles, the trial was halted due to this outcome. It was however found that the brain inflammation that arose was not due to the vaccine but rather due to an additive that was included to enhance exposure of the vaccine. No cognitive improvement was noticed in the subjects in the initial 1 year of follow up after the vaccines were stopped. However, something surprising was noticed when some of these subjects died and autopsies were done on their brains. It showed reduced numbers of SPs and infiltration of the brain with immune cells containing the β amyloid, meaning that the Aβ immunization stimulated the immune cells to clear away amyloid deposits in the brains of the patients. Additionally, some more remarkable findings after more years of follow up was that the progress of cognitive decline turned out to be much slower in subjects who received the vaccine. In conclusion, active and passive vaccination of Alzheimer's disease patients represents a very valid option for treatment and prevention of the neurodegenerative disorder. It can also be seen that results gotten in animals cannot always be extrapolated to be exactly what one would get in humans, a human trial is always necessary to ascertain the safety and efficacy of new inventions. It however seems certain that vaccines would increasingly become more main stream in the years to come for treatment and prevention of dementia as well as other neurodegenerative diseases.

CHAPTER 13

Pharmacological Products That Aid In The Prevention Of Dementia

Pharmacological agents for management of dementia encompassed in the latest protocols;

- **Cholinesterase inhibitors** are drugs which inhibit an enzyme that breaks down acetylcholine which is important for neurotransmission. It can be used to treat Alzheimer's dementia; mild – moderate type. Donepezil, Rivastigmine and Galantamine are well known examples and are approved pharmacological treatment options for the cognitive impairment in mild – moderate Alzheimer's dementia. Cholinesterase inhibitors efficacy has been clearly established in several short term (3 – 6 months) randomized controlled trials. Improvements were seen in the cognitive domains and global functioning of the subjects involved in these trials. There is some evidence that the beneficial effect of cholinesterase inhibitors can be noticed in the long term; up to a year. The drugs are available in easy to use forms such as oral and transdermal patches. Rivastigmine for example is available as a transdermal patch. A transdermal patch containing 4.6mg, 9.5mg or 13,3mg of rivastigmine can be used every 24 hours for treatment, the strength used should be based on the doctor's prescription. Patients may find the patch easier to tolerate as the degree of adverse effects of rivastigmine is lesser in transdermal patch compared to the oral formulation. This can be explained by the slower release of the drug through the skin. Adverse effects commonly noticed with the use of cholinesterase inhibitors are primarily cholinergic effects (diarrhoea, anorexia, weight loss, bradycardia, nausea, vomiting, and falls).The adverse cholinergic effects are more often dose related. They tend to disappear when the drug is released more slowly (i.e. transdermal patch) and with dose reduction. The most common adverse effects experienced with cholinesterase inhibitors are the gastrointestinal side effects.

- In cases of Lewy body dementia and Parkinson's disease, cholinesterase inhibitors (especially rivastigmine and donepezil) helps improve cognitive symptoms and it helps to stop visual hallucinations that may occur in this class of patients.

- In cases of frontotemporal dementia, **selective serotonin reuptake inhibitors (SSRIs)** and **trazodone** are found to be useful.

- In cases of moderate – severe dementia, cholinesterase inhibitors (donepezil) may be beneficial and should still be considered. After 3 months of stabilization of a patient with 10mg Donepezil, a high dose (11.5 and 23mg) extended release donepezil can be used for the treatment of moderate to severe dementia.

- **Memantine** is another drug. It acts by blocking a receptor in the central nervous system that is activated by glutamate. The glutamate neurotransmitter is a useful chemical in the brain that helps maintain our mood, helps us learn and maintain memory. The levels of glutamate in the brain are deregulated in Alzheimer's disease which interferes with normal function. The receptor that memantine acts on is called the NMDA (N-methyl D-aspartate) receptor. Memantineis beneficial in cases of moderate – severe dementia. Memantine can also be considered as a drug to be used for treatment of Alzheimer's dementia patients in situations where cholinesterase inhibitors should not be used or situations in which they cannot be tolerated due to adverse effects.

- A combination comprising of memantine and donepezil can be used for moderate –severe Alzheimer's dementia.

- A patient started on medications for dementia would require a follow up review after 4 to 6 weeks to check the adverse effects the individual is experiencing and hence adjust the drug dose as needed.

- A patient that is not tolerating a cholinesterase inhibitor even after dose reduction or slower titration has been done can be switched to another cholinesterase inhibitor.

- Memantine and acetylcholinesterase inhibitors could be used in cases of Lewy body dementia (DLB).

- Patients with cognitive symptoms in Parkinson's disease associated dementia can be managed with acetylcholinesterase inhibitors.

- In fronto-temporal dementia (FTD), neither memantine nor acetylcholinesterase inhibitors should be used.

- Supplements, herbal products and other pharmacological products are not recommended for the routine management of dementia.

- Atypical antipsychotics starting at low doses are the preferred pharmacotherapy for treatment of behavioural and psychological symptoms of dementia (BPSD). However pharmacotherapy should not be used as first line treatment. They should be used after non pharmacologic interventions have been attempted. They can also be considered if the symptoms are a source of distress to the patient or caregiver. They can be considered if it is contributing to a risk of harm to patient or others.

- Risperidone should be used for the treatment of agitation and aggression in patients with dementia. More novel evidence has shown that there is the possibility of using citalopram which is an antidepressant for improvement of patient's agitation when the symptoms are not severe enough to necessitate starting patient on antipsychotics.

- Dementia patients having severe psychotic symptoms and agitation may be given atypical antipsychotics such as **aripiprazole, risperidone, quetiapine** at a low dose.

- **Quetiapine and Clozapine** may be considered in people with severe psychotic symptoms and Parkinson's disease or Lewy body dementia.

- Management of mood symptoms and co-morbid depression can be done with selective serotonin reuptake inhibitors (SSRIs). Drugs should only be commenced after non pharmacologic therapy such as **cognitive behavioural therapy** (CBT), psychotherapy or reminiscence therapy has failed. Use of tricyclic anti depressants (TCAs) should be avoided.

- Acetylcholinesterase inhibitors should not be used in cases of vascular dementia.

- In cases of vascular dementia, cardiovascular risk factors need to be limited and cardiovascular or other systemic disease that puts the patient at risk needs to be treated in order to prevent vascular dementia. The primary prevention of vascular dementia requires treatment with medications for risk factors like diabetes, hypertension, dyslipidemia. For example, antihypertensive drugs have been proven to have a protective effect against dementia in patients. This is because a high risk of cognitive decline and stroke is closely related to elevated blood pressure that is left uncontrolled. Statins and omega-3 fatty acids as are further explained below are beneficial in maintaining cardiovascular health which can prevent vascular dementia:

  1. **Statins:** consumption of statins has been observed to be preventive for occurrence of dementia. Statins keep the cholesterol levels in the blood regulated. They maintain the integrity of the lining of the blood vessels.

2. **Omega-3 fatty acids:** observational studies and epidemiological studies suggest a protective role of omega-3 fatty acids against dementia in elderly who are cognitively intact. Features that may enable omega-3 fatty acids carry out this function include its anti-inflammatory, antiatherogenic, anti amyloid, antioxidant and its neuroprotective properties. The examples of omega-3 polyunsaturated fatty acids (PUFAs) includes the longer chain omega-3 forms like docosapentanoic acid (DPA), eicosapentanoic acid (EPA), docosahexanoic acid (DHA) which can be largely found in fish. It also includes the short chain omega-3 forms i.e. alpha linolenic acid (ALA), vegetable oils and nuts are good sources of this type. It is not clear as to whether or not consumption of the short chain form of omega-3 PUFAs is effective and opinions differ on that subject because ALA undergoes some processes in the body through which it

gets converted to the longer chain forms for use in the body. The effectiveness of conversion is affected by other dietary factors. For this reason the short chain omega-3 PUFAs effectiveness may differ from the long chains. The mechanisms through which omega-3 PUFAs exert its actions includes its protective role against cardiovascular disease especially with regards to inhibiting the formation of atherosclerotic plaques within the blood vessels as well as its role in reducing the risk of non-haemorrhagic stroke. Its work in improving cardiovascular system health is important as cardiovascular disease increases the risk of dementia especially Alzheimer's disease and vascular dementia subtypes. Long chain omega-3 PUFAs also produce cardiovascular health via antithrombotic and antiarrhythmic effects, blood pressure lowering effect, lowering of triglyceride levels, improvement of endothelial function. They also have anti-inflammatory effects that are beneficial in inhibiting the dementia process, the work by reducing the synthesis of pro-inflammatory cytokines, this helps subside the pro-inflammatory components of the disease process. Additionally, amongst the long chain PUFAs, DHA is an important component of the membrane phospholipids in the brain thus adequate omega-3 fatty acid levels in the body maintains the function of the neurons and may also protect against dementia by protecting the membrane integrity. Experiments in animal models show that when diet is enhanced with DHA, neuronal excitability is increased, neurotransmitter levels are improved and neuronal damage is reduced; this resulted into measurable improved memory performance noticed in those experiments. Lastly, omega-3 PUFAs play a pivotal role that is directly linked to the beta amyloid which is the hallmark plaque deposit seen in Alzheimer's disease. Omega-3 PUFAs enables its clearance from the brain and reduces its production from its precursor protein. Reduced risk of impaired cognitive performance is seen amongst populations that consume diets rich in omega-3 PUFAs and fatty fish. There is also an inverse relationship between risk of dementia and consumption of omega-3 fatty acid. Dietary consumption of fish is linked to a slower cognitive decline over time which is shown to be a complementary effect of omega-3 PUFAs as well as other nutritional components of fish. Omega-3 PUFAs are easily available as pharmacological products commonly made in form of oil capsules and syrup which can be prescribed for regular intake.

Other pharmacological therapies for dementia

1. **Biotin:** this is a water-soluble B-complex vitamin also known as vitaminB7.It helps the body metabolize fat, proteins and process glucose. The vitamin is an important component of many enzymes involved in metabolizing fats and carbohydrates; this influences cell growth and multiplication. Many enzymes of which it is a component process amino acids involved in protein synthesis. It has been previously known as co-enzyme R. Patients with dementia have been found to have low levels of biotin in the body. Unfavourable changes in the globus pallidus interna (GPi) and hippocampus which are both parts of the brain has been linked to biotin deficiency, those parts of the brain play important roles in subconscious movements and learning respectively. Deficiency of biotin causes dysregulation of the sodium dependent multivitamins transporter which is located at the

GPi and hippocampus. This is linked to those adverse changes that then occur. This highlights the need for biotin in prevention of dementia especially the Alzheimer's disease type. Biotin is needed to get needed glucose to the brain, so if it is deficient, the brain cells would not have sufficient glucose needed to function. It also enables insulin to function more effectively by increasing the sensitivity of tissues to it. Large doses of biotin; 100mg thrice a day is found to be neuroprotective. Biotin can be synthesised in our gut by intestinal bacteria, but it is not certain how much biotin is synthesised. Food sources with good content of biotin include beef or pork liver, eggs, yeast, whole wheat bread, avocado pear, salmon, cauliflower, cheese.

2. **Chromium:** Chromium exists in several forms, but the safe form is found naturally in many foods. The safe form is trivalent chromium and it is essential for it to be obtained from the diet because it serves several important functions in the body. There is a direct relationship between chromium blood levels

and cognitive function in the elderly. Higher chromium levels are associated with improved cognitive functions. Insulin resistance fosters the development of Alzheimer's-dementia and chromium enables better use of glucose in the tissues. Chromium helps overcome insulin resistance and aid cognitive function in elderly with mild cognitive impairment. Chromium is part of a molecule called chromodulin, this molecule helps insulin hormone perform its actions in the body which includes delivery of sufficient glucose to brain cells. Taking chromium supplements is necessary because absorption of normal dietary chromium in the small intestine is very low. Chromium picolinate is the form of chromium that is put in supplements, chromium is attached to three molecules of picolinic acid and this form of chromium is absorbed better. Improved learning, recall and recognition are demonstrated in elderly with dementia after supplementation with chromium.

3. **BF-7 silk protein hydrolysate and dementia (BF-7):** it was discovered by researchers that boosting the low levels of acetylcholine in the brain of a patient with dementia is pivotal to solving memory problems like having difficulty remembering faces, sluggish mental response and forgetting words the very time they are needed. So supplements are needed to boost it. The Brain Factor-7 (BF-7) is a derivative from silk protein that helps stimulate production of the acetylcholine needed to get your brain functioning normally without the memory problems aforementioned. The BF-7 is a rare substance found in the silk proteins of Korean silkworms; Bombyxmori. The BF-7 can pass through the blood-brain barrier. It also has neuro protective effects and aids restoration of cognitive functions.

4. **Sage leaf extract (Salviaofficinalis):** sage is used to describe a wise person and also is the name of this very wise plant. The plant is a perennial subshrub belonging to the mint family. It is a well-known spice used in the kitchen and has been long known

for centuries as a memory restorer. The plant produces its effect by cholinergic effects just as BF-7 does. It inhibits acetylcholinesterase thereby improving acetylcholine levels. It also improves mood and cognitive ability.

5. **Luteolin:** luteolin is a flavonoid that can be found in foods like oregano, green pepper, celery, broccoli, parsley, dandelion, thyme, chamomile tea, navel oranges, carrots, olive oil, peppermint, rosemary. It can also be isolated as a supplement and has been researched extensively for use in prevention of dementia. Luteolinis useful in prevention and treatment of Alzheimer's disease. It performs this role due to its anti-inflammatory activity. One of the major causal theories behind Alzheimer's disease is the amyloid cascade hypothesis. Many clinical trials have been done and attempts have been made to target this amyloid beta (Aβ) peptide but there is no single fail-proof treatment yet. This is because Alzheimer's disease is complex and the dementiais contributed to by several factors hence there is the

need for multiple therapies to be given to patients with dementia. Amidst this complexity, a consistent and quite prominent contributing factor to Alzheimer's is inflammation within the brain. Systemic inflammation also helps initiate Alzheimer's disease. This is where the importance of luteolin comes in by stopping inflammation. Luteolin also has a good antioxidant activity and can cross the blood brain barrier. The mechanism via which luteolin targets inflammatory processes and improves the outcome of Alzheimer's-dementia in particular still needs to be further understood but it does have beneficial effects in patients with dementia.

6. **Baicalin:** this is a scutellariabaicalensis root extract. Baicalininhibits beta amyloid aggregates. It interacts with copper and inhibits the formation of $A\beta - 42$ (AB1-42) aggregates. The AB1-42refers to one of the aggregate isoforms of the $A\beta$ protein that are formed in Alzheimer's disease. So once the protein aggregate formation is inhibited, the result is that Alzheimer's-dementia could be inhibited as

well. Additionally, baicalin inhibits oxidative injuries to the SH-SY5Y cells induced by AB1-42 aggregates. The SH-SY5Y cells are undifferentiated stem cells that can serve as a progenitor to some other brain cells; they can develop to other cells so they are very vital cells to be protected. Baicalin protects the cells by inhibiting H2O2 production which is increased when there is an accumulation of beta amyloid aggregates or a formation of plaques. This particular effect has been proven in research as baicalin has been shown to be important in regenerative medicine as it promotes differentiation of neuronal stem cells. Just by looking at these two functions alone, it can be seen that baicalin is a very valid supplement that can blunt the formation of plaques in the brain as well as inhibit their effects. It also shows that baicalin is a regenerative drug. This has the potential to modify the onset and progression of Alzheimer's disease markedly. It has been suggested through research as a possible drug for treatment of neurodegenerative disorders due to its proven regenerative effects.

7. **Resveratrol:** resveratrol has been shown to work as an; anticarcinogenic, anti-inflammatory, antioxidant. It is a drug that also gives cardiovascular and neurological protection. It is a polyphenolic compound (polyphenols are compounds that are mainly naturally occurring but also have synthetic /semi-synthetic derivatives, they contain the phenolring). Resveratrol is majorly synthesised from diverse plants in response to adverse conditions such as trauma, ultra violet light exposure, fungal infection. It is also commonly found in grapes and red wine. The neuroprotection effects of resveratrol have been observed in Alzheimer's disease, cerebral ischaemia, Parkinson'sdisease and even more recently in vascular dementia. It functions as a lipoprotein synthesis modulator which is protective against atheroma plaque formation and it inhibits platelet aggregation as well. These functions produce cardiovascular health and also

protect the brain simultaneously from vascular dementia and cerebral infarction. Chronic brain hypoperfusion resulting from occlusion of the major vessels that supply the brain can be prevented as well. Chronic brain hypoperfusion is a causal factor of cognitive impairment in ageing and neurodegenerative disorders. Oxidative stress which leads to release of reactive oxygen species and free radicals is limited in the presence of resveratrol. Brain blood vessels have a superior ability to produce high levels of superoxide compared to other vessels in the body, these superoxides can damage the nervous system and resveratrol is a potent antioxidant to blunt the production of such damaging free radicals.

CHAPTER 14

Latest Research/Clinical Trials On Dementia Prevention

There is a widespread interest in the field of dementia, numerous clinical trials are continually being carried out to find out new ways through which dementia can be prevented. Some of the latest clinical trials on the means of prevention are highlighted below:

Nutrition and Diet

Numerous clinical trials have been carried out on the role which nutrition has to play in the prevention of dementia. In a qualitative evaluation and systematic review of longitudinal and prospective trial, the effect of maintaining a mediterranean style of diet on the cognition of adults was evaluated. Roy Hardman et al found in this study that intake of mediterranean diets (this entails consumption of fruits and vegetables and a reduction in the amount of red meat, sugars and dairy products that an individual consumes) had a protective effect on the development of dementia. They found that individuals who adhered to this diet were found to have slower rates at which their cognitive functions declined and were even found to have improvements in cognitive functions as opposed to individuals who did not. The rate of decline and the improvement of cognitive function also correlated with the degree of adherence to the diet as individuals who were more adherent had better cognitive function compared to individuals who did not make as much use of the mediterranean diet. In the study "MIND diet slows cognitive decline with aging", Martha Clare Morris, S.D et al found that combination of the Mediterranean diet with the DASH diet helps to slow cognitive function. A combination of these diets was also associated with better cognitive functions than the use of the Mediterranean diet alone in some studies. Brain atrophy, one of the important hallmarks of dementia was also found to be slowed down when patients who had mild cognitive impairments were placed on a diet rich in folic acid, pyridoxine and cobalamin when compared with individuals who were placed in the placebo group in some studies. Recent studies have also shown that lower intake of saturated fatty acids was associated with better cognitive function later in life and as a result there is a resulting reduction in the risk of development of dementia. A recent meta-analysis of previously carried out research showed that a low serum level of Vitamin D was associated with a higher risk of development of dementia as it correlated with higher prevalence of dementia when compared with individuals with a higher serum

Vitamin D level. Vitamin D is known to serve neuroprotective functions by its action on the production of nitric oxide, an important neurotransmitter in the brain. It is also important for the production of nerve growth factor, an important factor that mediates the growth, proliferation and survival of neurons.

Physical Exercise

There is compelling evidence that physical exercise has a very important role to play in the prevention of dementia as has been shown by numerous trials. In one study, physical exercise was found to reduce the risk of cognitive impairment and dementia (particularly vascular dementia) independent of the age of individuals, their educational status or the presence of brain changes or other comorbidities. Another study found that individuals who engaged in physical activities had significant cognitive improvement which was more marked when physical activity was combined with some form of cognitive training: the duration of physical activity was found to be of more importance in reducing risk of dementia than the specific activity embarked upon as longer periods of physical activity correlated with higher cognitive improvements. Another study which observed patients over a period of eight years to assess the effect of exercise on cognitive function and risk of development of dementia found that the duration of physical activity was the most significant factor in exercise associated with a better cognitive function, with individuals who engaged in exercise for thirty minutes or more found to have a reduced risk of development of cognitive decline.

Modulation of Vascular Risk Factors

Vascular risk factors such as hypertension or diabetes can predispose to the development of vascular or Alzheimer's disease. As such, modulation of these risk factors aids in the prevention of dementia. There are a number of clinical trials and research projects that have been carried out to validate and assess this. A recent review revealed that proper management of hypertension with the appropriate antihypertensive medications, for instance results in up to a 55% reduced risk of cognitive decline, vascular dementia and Alzheimer's disease. The most effective of the antihypertensive agents in reducing the risk of dementia has been found mostly to be drugs which act on the rennin-angiotensin system of the body; a signalling pathway in the body that controls the blood pressure. Another vascular risk factor which can be modified to prevent dementia is dyslipidaemia. Some studies have found an association between the use of statins and a decreased risk for cognitive impairment as well as dementia. Appropriate management of diabetes has also been shown by recent research to be a good bet for prevention of cognitive impairment and dementia. Such studies have shown as much as a threefold increase in risk of development of dementia in diabetic individuals when compared with non-diabetic individuals.

<u>Stress</u>

Several studies have shown stress to be associated with a reduced level of cognitive function both by a direct effect and by the effect stress may have on other normal metabolic functions of the body. Some of these effects include inflammatory processes and changes in how the cells read the genes expressed in the brain. Such studies have thus gone on to show that proper management of stress can be an important tool in the prevention of dementia. A study found that meditation was associated with significant improvements in performance of individuals on intelligence quotient tests as well as tests of cognitive function, a major determinant of dementia. Another study assessed the flow of blood to the brain at the baseline points and after a period of meditation and revealed increased cerebral blood flow, thus suggesting that meditation has a role to play in the prevention of the vascular form of dementia.

<u>Immunomodulators</u>

Some clinical trials and studies have also looked at the role that substances which modulate the function of the immune system may have in the prevention of dementia. Some of the current modalities that have been utilised include immunisation with vaccines or antibodies such as tau peptide conjugate; the tau protein is a major protein implicated in the pathophysiology of dementia. In addition, some vaccines have been tried out in clinical trials to assess the efficacy in the prevention of dementia. Such vaccines include AN1972 and ACC-001, which were utilised to moderate degrees of success in the clinical trials. A more recent vaccine which is however currently still being tested in clinical trials is the AADvac-1 vaccine. Other immunomodulators that are still being investigated include aducanumab, crenezumab and gantenerumab. With further testing, the extent and nature of the role which these immunomodulators may play in the prevention of dementia will be determined.

Cognitive Retraining

Research on cognitive retraining is focused on activities which have been shown to increase the cognitive reserves present in individuals. The cognitive reserve entails the functional and structural alternatives that the brain is able to fall back on when pathological changes occur in certain parts of the brain. As such, even when the pathological changes that would otherwise lead to dementia begin to occur, the brain is more resilient and better equipped to prevent the onset of dementia due to these reserves. Studies have shown good educational and occupational achievements to be examples of activities that increase this reserve and as such, individuals with higher levels of academic and occupational achievement are more protected against dementia than uneducated or less educated ones. These achievements are even more protective when individuals keep at educating themselves into the later parts of their lives. Engagement in leisure activities has also been shown by some studies to aid the brain reserve and thus help reduce the risk of dementia. An important delineation made in the way cognitive training helps to prevent dementia and how physical exercise works as shown by studies is that while physical exercise has an effect on preserving the volume, structure and integrity of the brain cells, cognitive training improves the functioning and adaptability of the brain cells in the face of pathology With more ongoing research, more information on the concept of cognitive reserve would be unravelled which would lead to specific interventions that would help to preserve brain reserve, reduce the risk of dementia and prevent dementia.

Hearing Loss and Dementia

More recent research has identified hearing loss as a risk factor for the development of dementia. Hearing loss is of particular interest as it is a process which has been estimated to be present in as much as one-third of individuals who are above the age of 55 years. The exact mechanisms by which hearing loss causes dementia has not yet been fully described and there are more research projects being carried out on the subject. Current research data also has not clearly stated whether or not the use of hearing aids to correct the hearing loss improves the cognitive decline and this is still an area of ongoing research. Visual impairment is also receiving attention as a possible predisposing factor to the development of dementia and trials are being conducted to ascertain if there is any truth to this hypothesis.

Depression and Dementia:

Studies with long periods of follow up of patients have shown a link between depression and dementia, and even show a relationship between the number of episodes an individual has had and the severity of dementia. While research that has been carried out has not been able to confidently delineate between depression being a symptom of dementia or an independent risk factor, the latest studies indeed show that early identification and prompt treatment of depression when it occurs in any age group is associated with an improved cognitive function in later life compared to when depression was not properly identified or treated. Studies have shown a significant difference in the rate of cognitive deterioration in patient who were placed on antidepressants compared to patients on placebo treatment. The role of pharmacological and non-pharmacological managements of depression in the prevention of cognitive impairment and dementia is one which is still being actively investigated in order to ensure that more concrete evidence on dementia prevention is available.

Smoking

The latest research on the link between smoking and dementia suggests a very strong link between smoking and the development of dementia. Smoking causes dementia both by its effects on the vascular system and by direct harmful effects on the brain. Interventions to reduce and stop smoking have yielded a reduction in the development of cognitive function in the concerned individuals.

Social Contact and Isolation

Studies suggest that social interaction might prevent the occurrence of dementia, with recent research finding people who were unmarried or who lived alone at slightly higher risks of developing dementia. Research on the protective effects of being in close relationships, if any, continue to be conducted.

Brain Stimulation

Recent studies indicate that non-invasive means of stimulation of the brain, either by appliance of transcranial magnetic or electric currents may significantly improve cognitive function in healthy patients, thus helping in some form to reduce the risk of occurrence of dementia. In addition to this use of reducing risk in healthy patients, other studies have shown improvements in memory and cognitive function with brain stimulation in patients who already had mild cognitive impairment or early stages of dementia.

Pharmacological Clinical Trials

Another important area of consideration in the prevention of dementia is the role that some pharmacological agents may have in helping to prevent dementia. Some of these agents are those used in the modification of the vascular risk factors and have been shown to have some role to play. Some other agents which have also been studied also include cholinesterase inhibitors for which while the cholinesterase inhibitors have not been shown to generally reduce or prevent dementia, they have proven useful in specific individuals who express certain biomarkers not expressed in the general population, suggesting that the cholinesterase inhibitors interact with these special biomarkers in a manner that produces some protection. These results are slightly promising and continue to be evaluated in order to ensure that these relationships are concrete and based on good enough scientific evidence. Trials on the role of non-steroidal anti-inflammatory agents found that while prophylaxis with non-steroidal anti-inflammatory agents was not associated with significantly different cognitive function, it helped to reduce the rate at which individuals progressed to Alzheimer's dementia. This is as well still under further investigations. Ginkgo biloba was an agent which is being investigated for a possible role in the prevention of dementia. Many of the preliminary studies however seem to suggest, that there is no significantly important action of this agent in prevention of progression of dementia.

With many factors recognised as possible risk factors or protective factors, another area in which current research is being carried out is how a combination of these factors could serve more protective functions together as opposed to a single factor. In one such study, diet, exercise, cognitive training as well as management of vascular risk factors were combined against control groups and it was found that there was a slight improvement in functioning in these groups when compared with the control group. Another study failed to find any significant difference between two such groups and it is due to this that more research is still being conducted worldwide continuously in order to continue to find innovative solutions to the problem of dementia.

Summarily, dementia is a multifactorial illness, providing an avenue for medical personnel to work out means to modify and prevent its occurrence by thoroughly investigating the associated lifestyle behaviours or diseases. This is what births the latest and continual clinical trials that are conducted to find out how exactly these factors affect dementia and how the knowledge of this can be leveraged in order to come up with innovative and high impact means of prevention. While clinical trials in humans are generally faced with the problem of being able to accurately state whether or not an associated factor is responsible for the effects that are observed, with a higher number of trials that are conducted, scientists can make deductions more confidently based on the available data. As such, with more of these clinical trials and research projects would come more knowledge, arming physicians with power to prevent dementia now and in the future. The studies to date also almost seem to confirm the important role that the diet, physical exercise and modification of the vascular risk factors such as hypertension and diabetes have to play in the occurrence of dementia. Thus, these areas are the areas in which more research is needed and indeed in which more research is being conducted daily. As such, interventions on all of these fronts would seem to be of benefit in the prevention of dementia.

CONCLUSION

One of the major and complex brain functions of a human is cognition. The main cognitive functions the human brain performs are perception, attention, memory, motor skills, language and comprehension, visual and spatial processing and other executive functions. Each of these cognitive functions is controlled by different neuron networks located in various parts of the brain. Even the simplest daily activities require coordination of different cognitive functions. Hence, the quality of life of a human greatly depends on these higher and complex functions of the brain.

There are several medical conditions that can interfere with the good functioning of the brain and its cognition. Neurodegenerative disorders, heart diseases, vascular conditions, diabetes and many other medical conditions can promote cognitive decline.

Dementia is an umbrella term used to describe general cognitive decline in individuals due to different causes. The top most cause for developing dementia is recognized as Alzheimer's disease and secondly by vascular conditions. While some of these conditions are untreatable, there are certainly several risk factors that can be modified. Therefore, many research and studies approve the fact that dementia can be prevented or its onset be delayed by working on the modifiable risk factors. While the non modifiable risk factors are recognized as aging and genetic predisposition, the modifiable risk factors are known as physical inactivity, smoking, midlife hypertension, midlife obesity, diabetes, depression, low educational attainment, mid life hearing loss and social isolation.

The global as well as national costs in treating dementia and manging these patients carry a huge burden to the economy. In certain countries, Alzheimer's disease is in the top 10 list of diseases that causes death. The prevalence as well as the cost of managing this condition is predicted to rise in the coming years. Delaying onset of dementia by even for 5 years in patients reduced the healthcare costs in a greater manner. Therefore, WHO and countries unite together to improve prevention and early recognition of dementia.

Health experts call people into action by mentioning that several lifestyle changes could reduce the risk of dementia. These lifestyle changes are listed as smoking cessation, exercises – improving physical activeness, consuming diets rich in fruit and vegetables and fish (Mediterranean foods), avoiding obesity and diabetes, avoiding excessive alcohol intake, treating high blood pressure and lifelong learning/ cognitive training. Certain drugs such as antihypertensives, antidiabetics, lithium, steroid hormones and NSAIDs are believed indirectly promote risk reduction of dementia.

Research shows having a balanced diet that is rich in vegetables and fruits and low in calories are healthy for the brain. One of the highly discussed diets is Mediterranean diet which includes consumption of oily fish, olive oil, fresh vegetables and fruits, red wine and less amount of meat. The Mediterranean fish and olive oil are the main sources that bring Omega 3 and PUFA to the body. Omega 3 is involved in brain development, brain cell regeneration and improves the metabolic functions of the brain cells.

Similarly anti-oxidants are believed to deactivate the free radicals and protect the brain cells from oxidative damage. This is highly beneficial for the aging brain as the metabolism is sluggish at this state. Additionally, neurodegenerative disorders are also believed to be having a link with the metabolic dysfunctions of the brain cells. Consuming enough of antioxidants can help in this situation to scavenge the free radicals and to protect the brain from the active toxic substances produced during metabolic processes and thus prevent or delay neurodegenration.

Caffeine is another topic in discussion. Many studies identified caffeine to have a stimulating effect on the brain cells. The cell signaling and signal transduction were improved in individuals who consumed caffeine regularly. Also, the superfoods that are highly nutritious are believed to play a major role as well. Among the nutrients vitamin B group is regarded as vital as they have a direct link with the better functioning of nerve cells as well as regulating their metabolism.

Another diet that was highly discussed was ketogenic diet. This diet considers high consumption of fat, moderate consumption of proteins and a very low intake of carbohydrates. Although glucose is the main source of energy for the brain cells, glucose metabolism seem to impair with age as well as with neurodegenerative disorders and conditions like obesity and diabetes. During such a state the brain deprive of energy and the brain functions deteriorate.

This is when ketones come in handy. Ketones are products formed by fat metabolism. When there is a lack of energy supply by the use of glucose, ketones can act as the leading energy source and carry out functions of the brain similar and in an effective manner. Studies have found that ketones require lesser energy to enter the brain cells than glucose. Hence the energy need to process ketones is less and best fits for a brain that struggles with energy requirements. An increased level of plasma ketones increases the brain's affinity to ketones.

Ketones play a neuroprotective role using many mechanisms. The first and the foremost is by supplying abundant energy. In addition, ketones can also prevent pathological protein (such as amyloid) deposition in the brain cells that take place in neurodegerative diseases such as Alzheimer's disease. Ketones can also reduce inflammation by reducing inflammatory mediators and help reduce the risk of the same aforementioned brain conditions. Some studies show that these metabolic products of fats play a neurotrophic role and protect brain cells from damage. Altogether, by many roots and mechanisms, ketones reduce the risk of dementia. Therefore, using healthy fat sources such as coconut oil or ketogenic supplements are recommended as a step of prevention dementia and neurodegeneration.

Physical activities can improve the overall health and prevent health conditions that can cause dementia. Regular aerobic exercises that increase the heart rate are responsible in improving blood circulation and thereby reduce the blood cholesterol level, blood sugar level and tendency of clot formation. Hence the risk of diabetes, obesity, hypertension and stroke reduces which in turn reduce the risk of dementia. Improving the blood circulation to the brain is one of the best ways to supply it with enough energy and reducing toxic concentration of metabolic waste. That is how it helps in better brain functions and better cognition.

Involving in team sports, gym activities, group workouts can also improve social interactions. While social isolation is another risk factor of dementia, meeting people, making social relationships will help in sharing information, learning new things and using many of the cognitive functions of the brain. It is more likely training your cognitive brain and improving your abilities to learn, remember, focus, make decisions, comprehend and communicate.

Sex has a crucial role to play in the prevention of dementia. According to studies, cognitive function has a direct influence with the regular sexual activity, which is not only in the form of sexual intercourse but also included other forms of sexual activities. And men showed improvement in memory as well as executive domains of cognitive function, while women showed improvement only in their memory function.

Stress is a culprit of many unhealthy changes of the human body. Due to the chronic stress many people go through in the current years, millions of people suffer from obesity, diabetes, heart diseases and brain diseases. Dementia is also one of them. Chronic stress is believed to affect brain health in two main pathways; the first is by reducing the size of the hippocampus and secondly by increasing general inflammation of the body. Both of these changes promotes the shrinkage of hippocampus and precentral gyrus which takes part in cognitive processes such as thinking, memory, concentration and etc,. The best ways to handle stress is by involving in physical activities such as aerobic exercises, swimming, hiking and others that increases the level of anti-stress or happy hormone known as serotonin. Having regular sex, meditation, yoga, tai chi, spa treatments, acupuncture and many other relaxing methods and techniques can help you reduce the stress in your day to day life. Combating stress in an effective manner can save the hippocampus from shrinking by 2% that is believed to happen in chronic stress. This 2% makes a huge difference to the quality of life. By brain training and cognitive training a person can further improve 1% of hippocampus size.

Our hormones of the body have an important role to play in the cognitive function of the brain. The most important hormones that influence on the cognitive function are thyroid hormones, pituitary hormones (ACTH and Vasopressin), sex hormones (oestrogen, testosterone, DHEA and DHEA-S) and leptin. In elderly population, the age related sex hormonal decline and the following cognitive decline is evident. The use of HRT has a counter effect to increase the levels of these sex hormones as well as in improving the cognitive function.

Brain training or cognitive training is regarded as the way you could exercise your brain activities. Reading, singing, learning a new language or playing different mind games can be considered as cognitive training. Sudoku and the games that improve your thinking, memory and decision making processes are highly effective. Singing and learning music have also shown positive results.

According to studies, the other new ways of preventing dementia are by the use of Non-Steroidal Anti-Inflammatory Dugs (NSAIDs), Peroxisome proliferator-activated receptor (PPAR) agonists, Beta Amyloid (Aβ) Protein Aggregation inhibitors, neuroprotective proteins, Dimebon, conjugated estrogen and immunization.

Dementia cannot be treated in majority of cases. Therefore, managing its symptoms is regarded as the major aim in managing dementia patients. There are many therapeutic drugs such as cholinesterase inhibitors, selective serotonin reuptake inhibitors (SSRIs), trazadone, memantine and many others. Anyhow many supplements that can be added to daily diet are also regarded as helpful in improving cognitive decline. These supplements are Omega 3, Chromium, biotin, BF-7 silk protein hydrolysate and dementia (BF-7), sage leaf extract, luteolin, baicalin and Resveratrol.

Currently many types of researches and clinical trials are being conducted in the sole aim of finding different relationships between risk factors and dementia prevention. There are also several ongoing researches that are aimed at finding a treatment for dementia and the diseases that causes it. Anyhow, according to experts, the best way of handling this global health burden is by prevention or by delaying the onset of dementia symptoms, until the discovery of a treatment. This could reduce the healthcare costs as well as improve the health and wellness of general population.

REFERENCES

DANIEL AMEN, M.D, is the Founder and Medical Director of the Amen Clinics.

BENJAMIN ASHER, M.D., a board-certified New York City otolaryngologist.

DALE BREDESEN, M.D., a globally renowned expert on the neurodegenerative mechanisms of Alzheimer's disease. He has held faculty positions at University of California, San Francisco; UCLA; and the University of California, San Diego.

MICHAEL J. BREUS, Ph.D., is a Clinical Psychologist, Diplomate of the American Board of Sleep Medicine and Fellow of The American Academy of Sleep Medicine.

DONNA BROWN, M.S., is a clinical nutritionist in Connecticut. She is the Principal of Nutrition Kitchen LLC, her private practice dedicated to optimizing the health, lifespan, and vitality of her clients.

RICHARD P. BROWN, M.D., Associate Clinical Professor of University, is one of the world's foremost experts on the use of natural supplements.

Canada. Dr. Caplan worked for over 20 years at Women's College Hospital and is one of the few Canadian physicians board-certified in anti-aging and regenerative medicine.

DOMINIC D'AGOSTINO, Ph.D., is an associate professor at University of South Florida College of Behavioral and Community Sciences and its Department of Molecular Pharmacology and Physiology.

NORMAN DOIDGE, M.D., is the best-selling author of *The Brain's Way of Healing and The Brain That Changes Itself*, and a leading expert on brain neuroplasticity.

JOHN (JAY) FABER, M.D. is a clinical and forensic psychiatrist, child psychiatrist and adult psychiatrist at Amen Clinics.

VINCENT FORTANASCE, M.D., is a Clinical Professor of Neurology at Neurology Center in Arcadia, California. He is a board-certified Neurological Rehabilitation Specialist who has treated the Dalai Lama and Pope John Paul II.

MICHAEL B. FOSSEL, M.D., Ph.D., is regarded as the telomerase for cellular senescence in age-related diseases.

LEO GALLAND, M.D, a board-certified internist, is a Fellow of the American College of Nutrition and the American College of Physicians.

PATRICIA L. GERBARG, M.D., is Assistant Clinical New York Medical College. A graduate of Harvard Medical College.

DEBBIE HAMPTON writes about brain health on her website, The Best Brain Possible (www.bestbrainpossible.com). A survivor of severe brain damage, she describes the methods she used for a successful recovery.

RONALD HOFFMAN, M.D., Founder and Medical Director of the Hoffman Center in New York City, is one of America's foremost complementary medicine practitioners.

DAVID KATZ, M.D., the Founding Director (1998) of Yale University's Yale-Griffin Prevention Research Center and current President of the American College of Lifestyle Medicine.

JOSEPH MAROON, M.D., a world-renowned neurosurgeon and Medical Director of World Wrestling Entertainment and the Pittsburgh Steelers.

ROBERT MATHIS, M.D. is board-certified in Integrative Holistic Medicine, Anti-aging and Regenerative Medicine, and a Certified Clinical Nutritionist.

ALAN A. MAZAREK, M.D., is a board-certified neurologist and has practiced in Rockville Centre, Long Island for nearly 30 years. He has a strong interest in Alzheimer's Disease.

AARON P. NELSON, Ph.D., is chief of psychology at Brigham and Women's Hospital and an assistant professor at Harvard Medical School.

MARY T. NEWPORT, M.D., the author *of Alzheimer's Disease: What if There was a Cure?* helped to gain worldwide attention for the role of ketones in brain health.

PAUL NUSSBAUM, Ph.D., a board-certified Clinical Psychologist and Geropsychologist, specializes in Neuropsychology.

DAVID PERLMUTTER, M.D., is a board-certified neurologist and a Fellow of the American College of Nutrition.

FRED PESCATORE, M.D., is the Medical Director of Medicine 369 in New York, where he practices integrative medicine.

DALE PETERSON, M.D., is a past president of the Oklahoma Academy of Family physicians. An expert on iatrogenic illness (sickness caused by medical treatment).

MARY KAY ROSS, M.D., is the founder and owner of the Institute for Personalized Medicine in Savannah, Georgia.

PAMELA WARTIAN SMITH, M.D., is the owner and director of The Center for Personalized Medicine in Michigan. She is the author of *What You Must Know About Memory.*

JACOB TEITELBAUM, M.D., is a board-certified internist and nationally known expert on chronic illnesses. The author of numerous books, including *Real Cause, Real Cure.*

PART II

FREQUENTLY ASKED QUESTIONS ON DEMENTIA AND ALZHEIMER'S DISEASE

By

Selva Sugunendran

CEng, MIEE, MCMI, CHt, MIMDHA,MBBNLP, MABNLP

#1 Best Selling Author, Speaker & Coach

CONTENTS

30 Frequently Asked Questions:

1.

Who may be affected by Alzheimer's disease?

Given that Alzheimer's is a disease that can't be traced to a specific cause, we can only speculate on the combination of factors that make some people more vulnerable and likely to suffer from it. The following are some of the most common factors that need to be considered in order to evaluate the level of risk of an individual in case they are experiencing any mild symptoms, which could be completely unrelated to the condition in many situations.

The age of the patient

According to statistics, there will be about one person out of every 20 individuals over 65 years old who will end up developing the condition. The same statistics show that hardly a single person out of one thousand is ever going to develop the condition before they reach 65 years of age. This means that age is definitely a very important risk factor to consider.

A head-injured patient

Evidence has suggested that people who suffer from serious head injuries due to a strong blow are more likely to develop Alzheimer's. The risk is increased dramatically when the person who suffers from the injury is over 50 years old.

Heredity in some patient's families

This is also a factor that needs to be considered. There seems to be a limited number of people who inherit the disease from their parents, but there are many cases of people dying from Alzheimer's and their children not being affected.

The gender of the patient

Studies are also suggesting that women are more likely to get the disease than men are. The truth is that this is the least relevant of the factors that we have mentioned so far because those studies are still very far from conclusive.

Other probably factors to consider

There seems to be a link between education levels and Alzheimer's, but it's still too early to consider this to be a relevant factor to keep in mind. One thing that we can mention is that evidence is suggesting that people with a higher level of education are less likely to develop this condition than those with lower levels of education. This is known as mounting evidence, but more years are required to come up with a precise statement.

Anyone who is over 65 should be given an Alzheimer's test in case they start experiencing any symptoms just to rule out the condition or to be given proper care in case of a positive diagnosis.

2.

Signs & Symptoms of Alzheimer's disease

There are many reasons why people would consider going to the doctor when they feel their mental health is not optimal. The truth is that conditions such as Alzheimer's are not always going to be diagnosed if a person is forgetful or feeling disoriented at times, but there are some key signs and symptoms that people who are starting to develop Alzheimer's will generally experience. We are going to go over them so you can have a better idea of what to look for if someone you know is experiencing these symptoms.

Memory loss

This is going to be the initial stage of the condition is most cases. Memory loss can happen due to a large number of things, but frequent problems remembering things, and having to use reminders for things you used to remember on your own are usually signs of a problem.

Planning and problem solving

Simple problems that require the use of logic or mathematics might become challenging all of a sudden. If the problem happens once and it doesn't continue to happen, it will probably be an isolated incident due to being tired or many other factors, but a persistent situation with solving simple problems should be worth checking.

Forgetting how to get certain tasks done

If a person has specific daily tasks at home or enjoys playing a specific board game or card game,they will probably have no problems getting those daily tasks done or playing those games efficiently. If a person is developing this condition, they will have trouble getting those tasks done with the same level of ease as they once did. This would be a good time for an Alzheimer's test to be conducted in order to rule it out or properly diagnose it on a patient.

Being confused about the time or the location

Some people will start to feel like they have a very hard job keeping track of time. They will feel like a day already passed and they will get confused with dates. They might also start to feel forgetful about something as simple as knowing where they are headed when they start walking.

Having problems speaking and writing

When a person starts to have problems finding the right words to say during a conversation, or they feel like it's hard for them to write what they are thinking, they might also be experiencing early signs of Alzheimer's.

3.

Understanding signs and symptoms of Alzheimer's disease

Once an individual starts to show signs of mental abilities being lost and difficulty remembering things, this can cause serious concern in the person experiencing those symptoms as well as those around them. The symptoms are noticed by everyone who comes in contact with the person and this means that they will rarely let them go unnoticed or try to hide them because they cannot control when they will show those signs.

It's essential to seek medical attention and get a proper evaluation as early as possible in order to begin proper treatment. This is going to be extremely important because it will give people the time to adjust to the situation and take action. It's very important to understand the signs and symptoms that are often experienced when a person is going through the early stages of Alzheimer's disease.

The mild initial symptoms

The mild symptoms include forgetfulness and having a hard time remembering where you left your car keys and your sunglasses. This is often accompanied by having a harder time expressing thoughts with words and mood changes that happen for no apparent reason. This first stage is usually not going to be too much of a concern until the symptoms worsen and the person seems to be forgetting things quite frequently.

The moderate symptoms

Once Alzheimer's starts to cover more brain tissue, it will start to show moderate symptoms that can become extremely problematic for people. This includes memory loss that makes them forget how to get to places that they have visited frequently and difficulty carrying out tasks as simple as putting on clothes. At this stage, people might even have a hard time recognizing family and friends and it's quite apparent that they are no longer able to function as entirely independent individuals.

The most severe symptoms and stage of Alzheimer's

At this point, all of the symptoms that we have mentioned earlier become even more severe and the person starts to experience problems with the functions of their body. This means they will have a hard time swallowing food and keeping their balance. The progression takes about two years from the beginning stages of the severe symptoms until the person is unable to move efficiently and needs to be in bed all day long.

The progression of each stage will depend on the kind of treatment that is given to each person as well as their age and their general health.

4.

What actually happens to the brain over time when Alzheimer's disease progresses

There are many mysteries that surround the reasons why some people get Alzheimer's disease and why most people don't, but the condition is more common than most people imagine. Once it starts, it will start to attack the brain and deteriorate the mental health of the patient.

Being the most common form of dementia, this condition will progress to a fatal outcome even with proper treatment. The search for a cure or at least for a way to stop the progress of Alzheimer's is constant, but for now all we can do is give proper care to those who suffer from it.

According to research, Alzheimer's is caused by the abnormal buildup of plaques that get between the nerve cells in our brain. This creates a chain reaction that slowly destroys brain cells until the patient is unable to do anything on their own. The body will start to shut down slowly, but the progression is steady and impossible to stop with current medical treatments that are available.

The progression of the condition can begin even 20 years prior to symptoms that would prompt someone to seek medical attention for a proper diagnosis. Unfortunately, there is still no way to detect the early stages of the condition.

Once the mild and moderate stages begin, the plaques and the tangles will start to develop in areas of the brain that allow us to use our brains for thinking, planning and memory. That is the moment when people start forgetting things day by day and they feel confused and mildly disoriented. Once this happens, the personal and professional life of the patient will start to be affected and this stage can last as little as two years, but it could also take up to a decade to develop into severe Alzheimer's stages.

The late stages of the condition are terrible for the relatives of the patient because they will become strangers to the person suffering from the condition. They will no longer be able to take care of themselves properly and they won't even know how to get to the bathroom of their own home.

Once this stage sets in, the condition can last for up to 5 years on average before serious health complications set in and the patient needs to be hospitalized while being given proper care until their organs start to shut down completely.

5.

Communicating with your doctor about your ALZ disease

There is no question that being diagnosed with this condition is not an easy thing to experience. You will need to maintain a good line of communication with your doctor in order to ensure the best and most optimal treatments during the progression if the disease. Learning how to deal with this with a team effort mentality between you, your doctor and your family is the best way to approach this debilitating condition.

This is the main reason why anyone who is suffering from Alzheimer's should consider proper communication with their doctor while also consider taking other important steps to ensure maximum support. The lack of proper interactions between patients and doctors is going to have a very serious impact in the way that the condition is experienced and also in how long it can be kept from advancing to stages that will make the patient completely dependent on others.

We know that it can be stressful to even consider going to a doctor due to issues with memory loss and disorientation, but the sooner this stage is over with, the easier it is for a doctor to give the kind of treatment that will give the patient results they can trust. Remember that the earlier the diagnosis, the easier it is to plan ahead in every aspect of your life and in the prevention of an aggressive deterioration of your mental abilities. Some people with Alzheimer's are able to live relatively functional lives for well over a decade.

There is also the fact that medical advances are finally showing substantial results that might lead to a cure or at least a stop in the progression of the disease. This is going to make it a lot easier for people to handle their condition and maintain a good level of social interaction during the early and mid-stages of Alzheimer's, while also ensuring comfort during later stages.

Remember that doctor are there to help you move forward in life and to give you the kind of results that will help you live your life as normally as possible given the situation. There are plenty of treatments available right now to help people with Alzheimer's live their lives without serious concerns for a long period of time and this is the reason why you need to keep your communication with your doctor as open as possible.

6.

Diagnosing Alzheimer's disease

A series of evaluations of the symptoms the patient is experiencing will be conducted by a doctor and this is the most basic Alzheimer's test that leads to further testing. The first thing that the doctor is going to do is evaluate the earliest signs of the disease. This means looking for episodes of memory loss and impairment e.g. difficulty concentrating and finding it hard to locate certain places that the patient once knew how to find easily.

Other evaluations include the process of checking for language problems and changes in mood that come for no apparent reason and are new to the patient.

Distance distortion and not being able to drive properly are also common early signs that doctors will look for when evaluating and diagnosing Alzheimer's.

Another factor to determine the kind of testing needed from that point on is the age of the patient. Most people under 65 years of age are likely to be suffering from other not so serious conditions if they show these symptoms. Very few and rare cases involve people in their late 50's and anyone younger than that is extremely rare. The doctor is also going to evaluate your medical history to see if the patient has ever sustained any head injuries and if they have any other conditions that could contribute to those symptoms.

Interviews with people close to the patient are also going to take place in order to see the perspective of those around them. This is very important because the patient might not see things and remember them the same way that they do. Neuropsychological tests will always be part of the process too. Once those are done, a regular series of clinical exams will be taken in order to rule out any deficiencies and thyroid disorder, which can often be confused with the early signs of dementia.

In conclusion, there is no such thing as an Alzheimer's test in the sense that there are a series of tests that need to be conducted in order to reach a diagnosis. There is no single test that would help determine the situation so that a solid diagnosis could be provided. There are also many other conditions that need to be ruled out and this could make the process even longer. The results will then be used to conclude if the condition is indeed Alzheimer's in order to give the patient proper care for their condition.

7.

Preparing for the future during progression of ALZ disease

Alzheimer's is a condition that affects a large number of people all over the world and the need for proper attention, diagnosis and treatment is huge. This is not a condition that a person should experience on their own without any assistance. There will come a time when the individual who is suffering from ALZ is not going to be able to function independently and this is going to be extremely difficult to handle.

Being able to prepare for the future while the disease is still manageable and you have full mental capacity is going to be very important.

Contacting the official Alzheimer's disease organization in your area is going to be very important. The evaluation of each patient with this condition helps with the research for a cure. This does not involve taking part in any kind of experimental drug treatments, but it helps contribute important data that compares all kinds of factors that are very valuable to the medical community.

Once you have done this, you should make sure that you have a doctor that is able to take proper care of your needs. You might choose to continue treatment with the doctor that gives you the diagnosis of your condition, or you can decide to get someone else to see through your treatment in every stage of the condition.

You should also look for a counselor or psychologist because they will help you handle the situation and all of the emotional ups and downs that you will experience when you have Alzheimer's. This is very important and extremely useful because it will give you the chance to find comfort in their professional advice.

Get your personal life in order

While it's hard to even consider this to be an option, we need to act fast and get our life in order when it comes to 3 basic affairs. Our finances, our legal responsibilities and delegations and our medical care expenses. Once you are able to take care of those aspects of your life, you are going to have the required peace of mind to carry on with the journey of experiencing the stages of Alzheimer's without any other worries in your mind.

It's also important to handle those aspects of your life in the early stages of the condition because you might not be able to have the mental capacity to do this at later stages.

8.

The future outlook for Alzheimer's patients

There are many conditions and serious illnesses that we are fighting hard to eradicate. Cancer is one of the leading concerns worldwide, but Alzheimer's is definitely another huge problem and the way in which the person starts to slowly deteriorate and fade away is without a doubt something that no one wants to have to experience. The patient suffers in the beginning stages of the condition due to the progression of the limited mental skills and abilities, but then at the later stages of the disease, the condition greatly affects both the patient and those around them.

Aducanumab

This is an antibody that seems to be one of the most promising in stopping the progression of the condition, but there are a total of five DFA approved drugs that are specifically meant for Alzheimer's treatment and they seem to be helping people with temporary boosts in memory and thinking in general. The biggest hurdle with Alzheimer's research is the lack of federal funding for proper research, but there is also the fact that volunteers for clinical trials are not lining up to be used as test subjects.

It makes sense that people with this condition want to be cured, but they are also afraid of being subjected to clinical trials that could have serious side effects on their already weakened bodies and minds. This is one of the reasons why it has been so hard to be able to test the drugs properly and to go back to the drawing board based on results.

The amount of research that is done on this subject is going to be related to the kind of support that is given to the research. Many drugs are being developed that could help stop and even cure the condition, but this is not going to be easy and there is a lot of ground to cover. The only way that the research will be done with a more frantic pace is to raise more awareness about this illness and this is going to allow more chances for funding and donations to be given to the cause.

Alzheimer's is a very peculiar condition because of how it slowly robs the person of their independence and their ability to take proper care of themselves. Finding a cure for it needs to be in our list of priorities if we want results during all of Alzheimer's stages.

9.

Preventing Alzheimer's Disease

There are many mysteries that surround Alzheimer's disease and being able to prevent the condition is still not entirely possible. With that said, there are some important things that you can do in order to help keep your brain in top condition and this will reduce your chances of getting the disease. We are going to give you some important tips that you can implement in your daily activities to help you decrease the chances of developing Alzheimer's disease.

Your diet is very important

If you eat a lot of junk food and you don't consume nutritious foods that have all the vitamins and minerals your body needs, your immune system will be weaker and this is going to unleash a large number of health issues that could also contribute to suffering from Alzheimer's disease when you reach a certain age.

Eating more fruits and vegetables is going to be very important because your body needs proper nutrition instead of artificially flavored junk food or prepackaged TV meals that fill your stomach with chemicals and make you feel full, but your body is getting very little in terms of nutrients.

It's also important for you to increase the intake of Omega-3 fatty acids because the docosahexaenoic acid that is found in lean meats such as salmon and mackerel is known to lower rates of Alzheimer's. Taking supplements is also going to help and folic acid is one of the most useful and beneficial supplements for your body.

Exercise and meditate

People underestimate the value of exercise combined with meditation. The modern world is very hectic and even senior citizens are part of this fast-paced digital era now. We have gone from counting days, to counting hours just to get things done and even people who are retired are stressed and anxious because their children and grandchildren are always stressed and anxious.

Taking things easy and learning to live life without overcomplicating everything is going to be a great way to keep your body and your mind healthy. Stress is known for having serious effects on our physical health. Our bodies don't work at optimal levels when we are stressed and this lowers our defenses and hurts our immune system. If your immune system is compromised for long periods of time, you will get sick often and serious conditions can develop from this. Many of them contribute to the possibility of Alzheimer's in the future.

10.

Understanding Vascular Dementia

There are many causes for dementia. Vascular dementia is caused by a lack of proper blood flow to the brain and a large number of seniors are suffering from this condition all over the world. Just like all types of dementia, this type is gradual and it will start to affect the patient over the years. This particular dementia is the one that can be slowed down the most and people are able to live with it for over a decade in most cases.

There are many symptoms that have been linked to vascular dementia. One of the most common is that people are going to feel as if it has become harder for them to think fast and it seems like they are having a hard time organizing their lives and planning things out. Those symptoms are usually going to involve disorientation and confusion in many situations too and this is usually going to make the person feel concerned enough to visit a doctor for a diagnosis.

Another symptom will include difficulty keeping balance and walking. The truth is that all of these symptoms could be caused by many other conditions, but the important thing to keep in mind is that the combination of all of these symptoms will often lead to the diagnosis of some form of dementia. Not always, but quite often and it's even more likely that a form of dementia is involved if the person is over 60 years-old.

There are several tests that need to be conducted to determine if the person is suffering from dementia. Some of them include the proper assessment of their mental abilities with a series of psychological tests. There will also be a blood tests involved in order to find out if a person is feeling experiencing any kind of blood pressure problem. This can lead to the diagnosis of vascular dementias after MRI and CT scans have also been conducted to see if there is any damage done to the brain in any areas.

There are several treatments that can help a person live with the condition for much longer. Proper diets, weight loss, avoiding consumption of alcohol and tobacco and lowering cholesterol are all going to be extremely helpful factors that will help a person slow down the symptoms and the progression of the disease in a way that is considerably effective.

11.

Dementia with Lewy bodies

There are different types of dementia and this is one of the most common that can be diagnosed in people all over the world. The definition of dementia is given to all kinds of brain issues and gradual changes that damage functions slowly but steadily and the symptoms for each type of dementia are different.

The symptoms for this disease are hard to notice at first and they are known to affect all kinds of aspects of a person's life very gradually. This starts by making the person feel like they have trouble understanding things and even thinking about things they once had no problems analyzing.

These symptoms will gradually get worse and the concerns of the patient will become quite apparent. This is why reaching out to a doctor is important. It is worth noting that these symptoms could be due to a large number of issues unrelated to Lewy bodies dementia.

There will be times when the person is going to feel very alert and then they will be confused and sleepy with a lethargic feeling. All of these states will change through the day randomly and they will make the person feel like there is something different about their mood and behavior. This is usually the most common reason why men and women end up being checked and eventually diagnosed with dementia.

The tests that are given to a person to determine if they have Lewy bodies dementia are not specific and a large number of different tests are needed in order to come up with a proper diagnosis. There are brain scans that are often going to be seen as ideal for this diagnosis. The MRI and CT scans are amongst them and they will provide some signs and evidence that can lead to the diagnosis.

The treatments that can be given to people who suffer from Lewy bodies dementia are quite varied. None of these treatments will provide a cure for the condition, but they will help lower the severity of the symptoms until the condition reaches its most severe stages.

People who suffer from this particular dementia are known to survive for 5 to 14 years but some have been able to survive for much longer. It all depends on the kind of care that is given to these people and how they are able to handle and manage the condition.

12.

Understanding Frontotemporal Dementia

Out of all of the types of dementia that a person can suffer from, the frontotemporal condition is the one that can strike at the youngest age on average. There are people as young as 45 years-old who are suffering from this condition and it has been known to rarely affect people who are even younger. While most dementia cases of any kind are diagnosed at 65 or older, this type of dementia does have the highest rates of younger people who have been diagnosed with the condition.

This kind of dementia is like any other in the sense that it's also going to start developing slowly and it can take over a decade for the symptoms to reach critical stages. People will experience several symptoms in the early stages and they will eventually start to feel concerned and get initial tests done.

This includes behavioral changes that can seem to be selfish and very impulsive. There are also situations in which a person will experience extreme lack of motivation and difficulty handling social interactions when they once had no problem with them.

The person who is affected with frontotemporal dementia might also start to speak slower and they could feel like getting words out in the proper order could be difficult. This is often very frustrating and it contributes to the mood changes. Being easily distracted and having a hard time organizing and planning things will also be an alarm that something is not right.

There are also going to be memory issues but these are not as common in the early stages of the condition and they are more likely to be experienced after many years in the advanced stages of this particular dementia. A doctor will usually determine the stage of the condition after conducting a series of tests that are going to let the individual find out how they are feeling.

An assessment of the current mental abilities of the individual will be conducted with a series of tests and questions. Blood tests will also be conducted in order to be able to rule out any other conditions that might be causing these symptoms. The MRI, PET and CT scans can be a good idea in order to see what parts of the brain are being affected by the condition and in some cases spinal fluid might be removed to find out if the patient has Alzheimer's.

13.

Dementia is a Progressive Disease

Dementia progression is one of the most difficult things to witness for people who have relatives with this condition. It's a slow disease that takes a long time to affect the brain functions and it has very specific stages that need to be tracked carefully in order to provide the right kind of care to the patient.

Dementia is not always the reason why people are forgetful and they lose things easily. Some older people and even young people experience something called Mild Cognitive Impairment or MCI. This is not necessarily going to develop into Alzheimer's disease, but most cases of Alzheimer's are first diagnosed as MCI and then progress to the disease.

The stages of dementia

Mild dementia is considered to be the first of all dementia stages and people will start showing signs of it with short-term memory loss and misplacing objects often or having trouble expressing themselves. This could last a few years and in some people, it starts with a very mild case that can often be confused with MCI.

Moderate dementia will set in when the person is experiencing disorientation and might even feel like they don't know how to get to a location they already knew. Changes in sleep patterns are also common and personality changes can be noticed at this point as well. This is a stage of dementia that still allow the person to have full motor function, but the mental capacity issues start to be quite apparent.

The severe stages of dementia will start when people completely lose their ability to communicate with others and they will be unable to walk, sit, hold their own head up and even swallow. Then, the patient is not going to be able to control their bladder or bowel functions either and this leads to fatal complications.

Final thoughts

It's hard to say how long it takes for people to see this progression, but it can be years for the most serious symptoms to develop, but it can also start to advance fast depending on each person and their general health. It has been proven that a stress-free environment helps patients with dementia maintain a level of awareness and mental capacity for longer periods of time than those who are constantly stressed due to improper care. This is the reason why customized care plans for every patient with dementia are so relevant.

14.

Getting dementia help and advice in the UK

Being able to get the right kind of help and advice when it comes to dementia is going to be extremely important. Thousands of people are diagnosed with many forms of dementia in the UK each year and being able to find the right kind of guidance and advice is going to be essential. This is the reason why the Alzheimer's Society network has been created and you can reach them through www.alzheimers.org.uk in order to find out as much as you want about the problem.

The best thing about this particular organization is that they have a national dementia helpline for people who need advice on what to do. This is also meant to serve as proper guidance in case a person is experiencing symptoms and need to know where to go and what do to next.

There is also a huge community of people who share their experiences and connect with others. The best thing about this is that it provides a perfect support group of people who are going through the exact same thing. This kind of online community really helps those who feel alone and depressed because they will be able to find a large number of people who are also suffering from this condition.

There are many features that are also very attractive. People can volunteer to help those suffering from dementia and there is a support network that is constantly growing to provide the best possible service to anyone who requests help. Training is also provided to anyone who wants to learn how to take proper care of people who are suffering from dementia. This means that they will be given training that is going to help them deal with every stage of the mental deterioration that people with dementia experience.

This is definitely the kind of online platform that deserve to be shared with everyone you know. There is plenty of information available in the website and the community grows day by day. The support system and the encouragement for funding and volunteering is definitely to be considered more than enough to involve people in the process.

Be sure to let everyone know about this great and helpful website that is going to give a large number of people the hope and support they are looking for when dealing with this condition as patients or relatives of a patient.

15.

Guidelines for Advanced Stages of Dementia

There are many different factors to consider when a person is suffering from a stage of severe dementia and the kind of approach that is given to the care of a person at that stage is going to have a serious impact on the quality of life that the patient can expect to have. Knowing when the patient could be given medication for chronic conditions and understanding the risks and side effects of each of those medications is essential. This will allow the caregiver and the family of the patient to decide on which course of action to take in order to see the best possible results.

Some healthcare institutions and independent caregivers choose to use a holistic approach to alleviating some issues related to dementia, but those who are at a chronic stage of the disease are more likely to see no substantial comfort derived from this kind of alternative medicine.

The need for 24/7 nursing care is going to be determined by the inability that the patient has when it comes to taking care of their most basic needs. Not being able to feed themselves or not being able to use the bathroom without assistance are clear indicators that this person needs medical attention all day long and it should be seen as a priority to provide nursing care.

The use of antibiotics to take care of certain issues related to advanced stages of dementia is also going to be an important step in the treatment of the condition. Once an individual reaches the final stages of the condition, the need for proper treatment is going to be of paramount importance to alleviate the patient during those final stages of the disease.

Advanced dementia is to be considered a terminal condition and it needs to be treated as such. All of the care and treatment needs of a patient who is terminally ill are going to follow the same protocol regardless of the condition that is causing the terminal stage to begin to take place for any patient.

The substitute decision marker needs to be aware of the many decisions that need to be made at this stage in case the patient hasn't been able to leave all personal and financial matters resolved. The legal issues related to dementia patients should be solved as early as possible with the person still able to make decisions on their own when it comes to legal procedures.

16.

How Dementia Progresses and the Stages of the Mental Decline

There are many factors that need to be taken into consideration when the stages of dementia are determined and a time lapse can be provided. The truth is that all we have are average expectancies, but each person is going to be able to handle the condition with a varied degree of resistance to the mental deterioration. This is going to depend on how strong the person is and how good their physical and mental shape has been up to the point of the first symptoms being experienced.

There are several stages of dementia, but to classify them properly, the official number according to the global deterioration scale is of 7 stages. We are going to go over all of them, but officially, only 4 of these 7 stages are considered to be dementia.

Stage 1 is when a person is mentally healthy without any kind of issues. This means that they are not being forgetful in any way and they have no problems with their mental abilities at all.

Stage 2

Very mild decline in cognitive functions is found in stage 2, but this is still not considered to be dementia because many people tend to be forgetful and they often misplace items. This is something that a person can start to experience at some point in life but it will never progress to dementia at all.

Stage 3

This is the last stage that is not part of the dementia stages and it means that people might show a slightly higher level of forgetfulness and difficulty focusing and finding the right words to say. This is often due to nutritional deficiencies and stress. It might take about

7 years before this becomes a stage 4 and is classified as early dementia, but it could also stop there and never progress any further.

Stage 4

This is considered to be the first stage of dementia and it's the fourth stage on the list. When a person gets to this stage, they will have more frequent events in which their memory fails them and they will have a harder time managing their finances. They will find it much harder to complete tasks and analyze situations. Once this starts to happen the person might also stop socializing as often and they will experience a harder time managing their social life successfully because their memory loss will become an annoyance to them and to those around them.

Stage 5

This is basically the next level of severity of the same symptoms that have been experienced during stage 4. This means that the frequency of the forgetfulness and difficulty articulating words will be increased.

Stage 6

The severity in this stage is much higher and the patient is no longer going to be able to remember a lot of information about their past. They will start being delusional and their sense of orientation will be badly damaged to the point of needing someone to guide them back to their own homes.

Stage 7

The person is no longer able to control basic body movement and will need to use a wheelchair. Even the most basic activities such as using the bathroom and speaking will become extremely difficult.

17.

How to improve healthcare for those affected by Dementia

There is no way to deny that the biggest issue that we are facing right now when it comes to dementia treatment and healthcare, is the lack of awareness of the condition. Everyone has heard of Alzhemier's at this point, but the word dementia is often misinterpreted by people and linked to deranged and violent individuals who are in straightjackets.

Dementia is a very complex disease that will start to attack the brain quite slowly. There are many types of dementia and Alzheimer's is one of them, but the average individual out there has no idea about this and would never associate Alzheimer's with the word dementia. This is mainly due to the lack of proper campaigning to increase the awareness of this terrible illness.

The biggest problem that people with dementia are facing is that healthcare options for this kind of condition are very expensive due to the intensive care that is required when the disease reaches an advanced stage. Some patients might need 24/7 assistance for the last 4 to 6 years of the condition and this is combined with the need for expensive treatments that are often going to require changes in prescription and proper monitoring.

The best way to improve healthcare for dementia is to get more people to see how important it is to find a cure for it. The main hurdle for dementia is that it will never get the level of priority that is given to cancer or heart disease because it's considered to be a disease that only the elderly suffer from. This is true for the most part, but some people are diagnosed with the condition as early as their late 50s and this means their lives are completely halted by the condition.

The future for Alzhemier's treatment is looking good, but there is no cure for this condition at this point. Available treatments help delay the symptoms of brain function deterioration, but the outcome is still inevitably fatal with the current findings and treatments.

If you want to learn how to help support and reinforce the research and healthcare options for this condition, we suggest that you check out all of the available information found here. You can also get involved by being an active contributor in social media. You can post information on dementia and give people important data. This will help them see just how important it is to take proper care of people who suffer from this condition.

18.

In search of Dementia Treatment

There is no question that a search for the cure to dementia is always an important part of the battle between medical science and the conditions that we are unable to cure. Most forms of dementia can be slowed down in order to allow the patient to live for at least 10 to 15 years, but all that has been done with current medicine and treatments is lower the symptom intensity for a few extra years, in order for the person suffering from dementia to be as independent as possible.

The most important aspect of the research for proper dementia treatment is that more people need to contribute to the studies and testing by volunteering to get medical assistance with experimental drugs and treatments. Unfortunately, the very nature of allowing this kind of testing to be done is a huge risk for the patient due to the unknown outcome of those treatments.

The good news is that most of those experimental treatments have allowed doctors to find new treatment options that have been quite successful in slowing down all kinds of dementia, but the idea is to be able to find a cure, or at least slow the progress down at such level that the patient survives the disease by dying of old age before the symptoms become unmanageable.

Increasing awareness of this condition is also going to be very useful and this is going to help determine how much success comes from it. Social media has played a major role in helping raise funds for the cure of dementia and for better treatment options to be given to people who are still in their early senior years and want to be able to live their late years peacefully and calmly.

There is still a lot of road to cover if we are ever to be able to handle this kind of disease. There is nothing more important and valuable than being able to find cures for conditions that have been a burden to humanity since the very beginning, but the truth is that in order to make that happen, we need to make sure that we can get as many people involved and as much funding as possible can be raised for this purpose.

The idea is to be able to eventually reverse and cure the disease and then we will no longer just be looking for ways to slow it down.

19.

Stress and How it Damages the Brain

We live in a society that seems to be perfectly fine with the idea of being stressed out all the time. We feel like we are going to develop a great deal of resistance to the feelings of stress and that we can handle them as often as needed. The problem is that the complete opposite happens with stress. We don't get used to it and we don't develop any kind of resistance to it. Instead, it starts to damage our brain slowly, but steadily.

The constant spikes in our levels of cortisol are going to end up taking a very serious toll on our physical and mental health. There are plenty of studies indicating that chronic stress is highly related to a large number of mental disorders including anxiety, depression and even dementia. This is a serious cause of concern due to how stressful our lives are in modern times and how little time we have to relax and get rid of that stress.

Stress can lead to brain shrinking as it starts to reduce the volume of gray matter inside our brains. The most affected regions are often those that control emotions and physiological functions in general. There is also proof that shows how a very stressful event can lead to brain cell destruction. This means that people who suffer from a great deal of emotionally stressful situations are more likely to end up suffering from a mental condition.

The memory is also going to be highly affected when we are in constant stress. Even worse, the amygdala that is responsible for the processing of fear and fight or flight emotions is constantly triggered even when no serious threat is around and this means that we are in a constant "survival mode" that is taking a very serious toll on our bodies in every possible way.

The best way to avoid this problem is to learn to meditate and to find the time to relax after a hard day of work. A stressful work environment requires that we learn proper time management in order to ensure that we are able to relax after the hard work is over. Exercise, meditate, spend some quality time or even a few laughs with a friend or family member, but whatever you do, you need to make time for your personal relaxation or you will end up with accumulated stress that is very harmful to your health.

20.

Understanding signs and symptoms of Alzheimer's disease

Once an individual starts to show signs of mental abilities being lost and difficulty remembering things, this can cause serious concern in the person experiencing those symptoms as well as those around them. The symptoms are noticed by everyone who comes in contact with the person and this means that they will rarely let them go unnoticed or try to hide them because they cannot control when they will show those signs.

It's essential to seek medical attention and get a proper evaluation as early as possible in order to begin proper treatment. This is going to be extremely important because it will give people the time to adjust to the situation and take action. It's very important to understand the signs and symptoms that are often experienced when a person is going through the early stages of Alzheimer's disease.

The mild initial symptoms

The mild symptoms include forgetfulness and having a hard time remembering where you left your car keys and your sunglasses. This is often accompanied by having a harder time expressing thoughts with words and mood changes that happen for no apparent reason. This first stage is usually not going to be too much of a concern until the symptoms worsen and the person seems to be forgetting things quite frequently.

The moderate symptoms

Once Alzheimer's starts to cover more brain tissue, it will start to show moderate symptoms that can become extremely problematic for people. This includes memory loss that makes them forget how to get to places that they have visited frequently and difficulty carrying out tasks as simple as putting on clothes. At this stage, people might even have a hard time recognizing family and friends and it's quite apparent that they are no longer able to function as entirely independent individuals.

The most severe symptoms and stage of Alzheimer's

At this point, all of the symptoms that we have mentioned earlier become even more severe and the person starts to experience problems with the functions of their body. This means they will have a hard time swallowing food and keeping balance. The progression takes about two years from the beginning stages of the severe symptoms until the person is unable to move efficiently and needs to be in bed all day long.

The progression of each stage will depend on the kind of treatment that is given to each person as well as their age and their general health.

21.

The survival trends for people with dementia

Just as it happens with the predictions in terms of the incidence of dementia, the survival trends are going to be linked to the number of people who are able to get proper care and the latest medication available to treat the condition. This means that we can predict a higher number of survivors that will manage to die of other old age related conditions while they are receiving treatment for dementia. It's also important to consider the fact that most people will start suffering from dementia at no less than 65 to 70 years of age, so this means that many of them could die of other conditions before dementia is to blame for their passing.

There is no way to deny that we have a large number of diseases to deal with. Some of them have more funding than others and some of them have more support and awareness to back their research up. The important thing to keep in mind is that dementia is a very serious condition that affects a large number of people. The condition slowly deteriorates the brain and many individuals will suffer from it. The condition is emotionally taxing for the patient as well as their loved ones due to how they will eventually even forget who their closest family are and where they live.

The survival trends are looking quite optimistic for developed countries. This is mainly due to the latest medication available, which is extremely expensive for people who are on basic healthcare in their countries or people without insurance. The biggest concern for many of these individuals is that they are likely to have no proper care for their condition and this will cause far faster deterioration of the brain.

It has been proven that the simple idea of being tolerant and understanding with a patient that is suffering from dementia is going to be extremely helpful. Stress has been heavily linked to dementia and once a person is suffering from dementia, higher stress levels are going to contribute to a faster deterioration of the brain.

It seems like developed countries have the advantage of being able to provide better care for people, but the highly stressful modern life is not helping matters even for those who are financially stable. The one factor that is very important in a good economy is that people are more likely to have better dietary habits and to become aware of the need to engage in proper time management to lower stress levels.

22.

Understanding Diagnosis and Treatment of Dementia

One of the best ways to help treat any kind of condition is to see what works and what seems to provide no visible results. This means that healthcare facilities need to constantly monitor the quality of life and the progression of each patient with dementia. This needs to be paired up with the kind of experiences that they have with specific medication and treatments that might be enhanced or discarded for future treatments.

The biggest hurdle for dementia care is in the lack of awareness of the condition. Studies show that most people out there don't even know about dementia until someone they know is suffering from the condition. This is not the case with a disease such as cancer because everyone hears about it or knows at least one person who has died of cancer or suffered from it.

One problem with dementia is that proper diagnosis and care for the condition is extremely expensive when compared to other conditions. The process of diagnosis is very tedious and complicated as there are several tests that need to be conducted in order for the condition to be properly diagnosed. This leads to a very frustrating situation for those who don't have insurance that covers this sort of testing.

The social care aspect of dementia is still quite bad in most countries. There are some regions of the world that have proper dementia healthcare facilities that also provide social care and help keep the patients socially active. This is a great way to help them feel happier and to avoid faster mental deterioration due to feelings of frustration and stress.

The treatment coverage needs to branch out and look at people with dementia based on the kind of treatment level they get. There are those who have dementia and have received a conclusive diagnostic. Then you have those who are not diagnosed and still untreated. The other group is those that have been diagnosed but they are not receiving treatment for a number of reasons, and then you have those who have been receiving care since their diagnosis.

Those who have been getting proper care need to be divided between those who are getting acceptable outcomes in the quality of life they have during the condition and those who don't. That is going to reveal what kind of treatment variations work and which ones are not so successful.

23.

Assessment & Planning of Care for those affected by Dementia

Dementia is a very debilitating illness that is not reversible and there is still no cure for it. However, there are ways in which we can help people who suffer from this kind of condition maintain their way of life and that allows them to keep their dignity as much as possible. If certain needs are met, the person affected by dementia is going to be able to live in a safe environment that suits their condition and their limitations.

Proper assessment of the condition is necessary

The treatment for dementia is going to depend on the stage of the condition and how much of the brain has deteriorated because of it. The kind of care that is given to a person on the initial stages of the illness is nothing like the treatment that is given to those who have been suffering from it for a long time.

This is the main reason why the proper evaluation of the condition is essential and tracking its evolution is going to be just as important to make necessary changes in the way that the patient is cared for and treated.

Individual care planning

Every person who suffers from dementia experiences different problems, but most stages have a large number of symptoms that are commonly displayed. With that said, the need for individual care planning is very important and no two patients are going to have the same kind of care given to them.

The process of creating a customized care plan for a patient is going to be determined by their symptoms and their most common reactions when they feel lost or they feel their cognitive skills are failing to help them get through the most common problems.

Family members and friends should be involved

Every person that interacts with the individual that is suffering from dementia should be involved in this process. The ideal situation is for everyone around the patient to know how to deal with any kind of problems and issues that relate to dementia. This is going to create a much better environment for the patient.

Anxiety, depression and a wide range of emotions including anger and indifference are all going to be experienced by people with dementia at some point during the progression of their condition. The best way deal with this is for everyone to be as informed as possible.

24.

How can you take care of a person with Dementia?

This is a very common question and the truth is that there is no easy answer for it. There are all kinds of problems that people face when they are dealing with dementia. A caregiver needs to be prepared for several stages that the patient will experience. This is one of the reasons why health care professionals are often trained in dementia care exclusively because this helps them provide the best possible care to their patients.

The first stage

People who are in the first stage of dementia are often going to experience symptoms that they can handle on their own. They are still going to be able to take proper care of themselves during this stage and they will only experience mild memory loss and orientation issues that clear within a few minutes. This is typically a situation that requires no assistance from people, but it would be good for a doctor to start evaluating the patient and keeping track of their progression with the condition.

The second stage

This is going to require assistance because the person is going to start experiencing serious memory loss and they can start to feel lost when driving in the streets and when trying to locate an area that they have visited many times in the past. This is one of the most serious concerns that people experience when they reach this particular stage and that is one of the reasons why it is recommended that they don't go outside without a caregiver or at least with a friend or family member.

This is also a stage that is going to make the person feel extremely frustrated because they won't be able to handle their lack of ability to perform tasks that they once found to be so simple and easy to do. Emotional and psychological support will be very helpful during this stage.

The third stage

This is going to be a difficult stage because the person is no longer going to be able to do anything without assistance. They will lose their independence for the simplest activities and they will need a professional caregiver to help them with everything they need to do.

This is one of the reasons why patients on the later stages of dementia need to be in bed or using a wheelchair most of the time. They can't communicate properly and they even have trouble eating without assistance.

Caring for patients with Alzheimer's is a huge contribution to help those in need while a cure is found for this debilitating and fatal condition.

25.

Looking after a Patient with Dementia

Taking proper care of a person who is suffering from dementia can be a very difficult process. All dementia stages have their own unique set of symptoms and the kind of care that is given to people during those stages is going to depend on the severity of the problem. Some people experience certain symptoms earlier than expected, while others maintain their mental health for longer than most medical records would expect and suggest.

Once a person has reached stage 2 of dementia, they need to be given more attention and someone should be able to keep an eye out on them in case they get seriously disoriented and lost. Once the patient has reached an even higher level and gets to stage 3 of the condition, they will need to be taken care of all day long as even the most basic activities will prove to be impossible for them.

Hobbies and interests

The process of dementia will slowly make the person incapable of working in any kind of profession they once knew, but they can still maintain a good level of interest in hobbies as it is easier to retain that kind of information. This is one of the best things that any caregiver can do in order to help a patient that needs to stay busy and maintain the best possible level of mood and spirits during the progression of the condition.

Get family and friends involved

It's always important for a person who suffers from Alzheimer's to be able to feel as normal as possible. Interacting with friends and family in activities that don't require too much thinking can be a great way to help a patient feel relaxed and experience happiness during those moments. This has been proven to help them slow down the deterioration of their brain.

Taking care of the bedridden

When dementia reaches the final stages, the person is no longer going to be able to stand up, walk, sit, or even hold their own head up straight. This is the stage of the disease that requires attention from a nurse in most cases and the patient will need to be fed and cared for completely.

It's important for patients with dementia to get the help they need and the assistance that will make their illness more bearable as it moves from one stage to another.

26.

The importance of palliative care for dementia

Dementia is still a disease without a cure and this makes it an extremely difficult thing to deal with. Proper healthcare for dementia is known as palliative care because what it does is help the patient live with the condition with as much comfort as possible. There are several factors that are needed in order for treatment to qualify as palliative and we are going to go over the basics.

The main goal with palliative care is not to rush or to halt the progress of the condition, but to simply ensure that the person who is suffering from it is going to be able to live the remaining years of their lives without any serious discomfort.

It's also important to establish care planning in order for the patient to be able to let the caregiver know his or her wishes once he condition deteriorates all brain functions and makes it harder for the patient to be able to make decisions as the condition worsens. The best way to handle this kind of situation is to make sure that the patient is able to leave specific instructions of what should be done in regards to their assets and once their mental abilities are no longer optimal.

There should be a formal nomination that gives a person the rights to make financial and personal decisions for the patient in case they didn't leave any specific instructions in any given scenario. This is why it's encouraged for them to make sure that the can provide as much detailed instruction on their wishes before they reach that stage of dementia.

Evaluating the capacity to make decisions

When a person is suffering from a highly debilitating condition such a dementia, they are going to be evaluated by a professional in order to see how their decision-making capacity is doing as the condition moves forward.

In order for someone to qualify as mentally capable, they need to be able to understand all information that is relevant to any decision-making process. They should also be able to retain any kind of information for long enough to make decisions and they should be able to make this decisions without any external influence or coercion.

In conclusion, palliative care and everything that goes along with it is very important for dementia. This is going to help establish a huge difference in the kind of life that people can expect to have when they suffer from dementia.

27.
(TO ADD MORE STATISTICS)

The Impact of Dementia Worldwide in 2015

It can be quite hard to see how little information is out there for those who have never experienced dementia in their social circle. The truth is that never being affected by this disease is just luck of the draw. The statistics on the number of people affected globally is truly alarming and it reminds us of the importance that comes from proper education in regards to this terrible condition. Let's now look at some global statistics that are undeniably relevant and hopefully they will help raise even more awareness on the subject.

In 2015, the number of people who suffered from dementia all over the world was over 9 million. This means that one person every 3 to 5 seconds was diagnosed with the condition. The biggest concern is that the numbers keep climbing higher every year and there are close to 47 million people living with this condition right now. The increase in dementia cases will rise even more in low to middle-income countries due to how much the general wellbeing of an individual is involved in the possibility of having dementia after 65 years of age.

The regions with the lowest number of research facilities that are entirely dedicated to dementia include Africa, Central Asia, Latin America and Eastern Europe. It makes perfect sense that the poorer the country, the harder it is for proper dementia care to be found. This is a condition that is considered to be a disease of the elderly and the priority in developing countries is to use the scarce funds and recourse to treat diseases that attack people of all ages.

There is also an obvious issue with the number of health care professionals that are specialized in the treatment and care for patients that are suffering from dementia. This lack of professional care and the little priority given to the condition makes it even harder for people to get help. There is no estimate time for this to improve in smaller countries, but as long as the economy is in bad shape, the treatment for dementia will remain as a secondary concern.

The incidence of dementia all over the world is considerably large in 2015 and it has been larger than in previous years. The number of people who go onto the internet and search for dementia and Alzheimer's symptoms is also growing all the time.

28.

Important Facts About Dementia in 2016

There are many studies and research campaigns that have been conducted in order to help shine a brighter light on the condition that we know as dementia. We are going to be talking about some of the most important facts that people should know about and how they are affecting the world of dementia care and treatment.

Support for dementia healthcare systems

The first fact to consider is that a smaller level of attention is given to services and centers that are dedicated to the treatment of dementia. This makes perfect sense as there are many other conditions that can be considered more important and relevant for a number of reasons, but the need for more awareness and relevance is huge if we want to see any serious improvements.

Diagnostics coverage

The coverage that is given to proper diagnosis for dementia is quite low. The number of people living with dementia with proper diagnosis for it is as low as 40%. The reason why this happens is because dementia is a very complicated disease that cannot be diagnosed by a single test. There will be blood tests, physical tests and psychological tests that are going to have to be conducted in order for anyone to be successfully diagnosed.

The cost of many of those tests is quite high and this is one of the most compelling reasons why you are very unlikely to see them as part of any basic health coverage plan.

Specialized care is underdeveloped in most countries

There has been an increase in healthcare centers that specialize in dementia treatment, but this is only seen in developed countries. It's very rare to hear of any institution that is specialized in this kind of treatment if the country is experiencing any kind of crisis in the economy. The budgets for medical facilities and staff is usually assigned to conditions that affect a larger number of people of all ages and this kind of priority is logical, but not optimal for the fight against dementia.

Health care funds distribution does not see dementia as a priority. It's hard for a disease that only affects the elderly to become a priority amongst other conditions that are known to affect people of all ages and demographics. The only way to increase funding is to increase awareness so that those who support priority conditions will also consider contributing to the treatment and cure of dementia.

29.

Possible Trend Shifts in the Future of Dementia Incidence

While it can be hard to predict what the immediate or even long-term future is going to be like for dementia, we can already see the possibility of certain things changing. For example, a decline in the incidence of dementia for people between 65 and 70 years of age is a possibility. This is mainly due to a more adequate lifestyle and diet that is the direct result of a social environment that is much more aware of the importance of being healthy and fit.

There are many studies that are leading to the direct relationship between dementia and alcohol or drug abuse. The same goes for tobacco consumption and for poor eating habits. A sedentary life and lack of motivation and drive in life have also become important factors to consider. This is mainly due to the large number of dementia patients that have reported substance abuse of some kind.

Obesity and high cholesterol are also linked to this condition and the number of people with dementia who have at least one of those problems and history of dietary neglect or substance abuse is quite convincing. The one thing that we need to consider is that developing countries are more likely to have a large number of people who have poor dietary habits. The poorer the region, the harder it is for people to consume healthy foods on a daily basis. Also, the lower the economy, the higher the chances that people will engage in drug or alcohol abuse.

These are all factors that could determine the incidence of dementia increasing or decreasing in some regions. The more developed countries have a lower number of dementia patients when compared to countries that are still developing or currently suffering from a serious financial crisis. Healthcare is extremely scarce in places where more pressing concerns are prioritized.

This is a fact and it will never change. It takes us back to the way society works with everything else. Things that are considered a norm of developed countries are not important or relevant in countries that are facing any serious crisis. If we are to predict the future of dementia incidence, we need to look into the future of each region and country individually for the answers. The best way to ensure a good future is to continue to raise awareness of the condition.

30.

The Global Cost of Dementia Treatment

The levels of awareness for dementia care and treatment is still quite low when compared to other conditions and diseases. This is to be expected based on the economy of each region, as conditions that only affect the elderly are more likely to be seen as unimportant when compared to other conditions that affect a large demographic. With that said, the global expenses that are related to dementia are on the rise.

The cost has increased from $600 billion in 2010 to $800 billion in 2015. This means that there is an incredibly large number of people who are suffering from the condition and being treated for it. The regional distribution costs for treatment have increased steadily in every region and the need to increase awareness in order to get more support is huge. The global costs of treatment would be fine-tuned if awareness was widespread, but this continues to be such an unknown condition, that most people only know of Alzheimer's and have never even heard of any other form of dementia.

The lower the income in any country, the harder it will be for proper care to ever reach those areas and the available care is extremely expensive for a person with an average job and salary. The prevalence of dementia is going to be determined by a large number of different factors, but the truth is that the countries facing the biggest challenges are the ones that have the lowest income rates.

The costs of dementia treatment are only going to continues to rise all over the world. This will happen as more information is made available on the internet and a larger number of people are diagnosed after they review symptoms online and decide to get checked. Many individuals living with dementia are unaware of the problem until their brain deterioration reaches alarming levels.

The life expectancy of an average individual worldwide is rising, but conditions like dementia are slow acting diseases that could take 10 to 15 years to fully develop into a fatal outcome. This means that the average life expectancy in some regions is 75, but a diagnosis of the condition usually comes between 67 and 70 years of age, which means the person will not die from dementia, but of other health issues. The problem is that it's still very hard to tell just how much of an influence dementia has on other conditions.

www.ingramcontent.com/pod-product-compliance
Lightning Source LLC
Chambersburg PA
CBHW061743250726
48657CB00001B/16